THE ULTIMATE Gout Diet Cookbook For Seniors

Low Purine ingredients

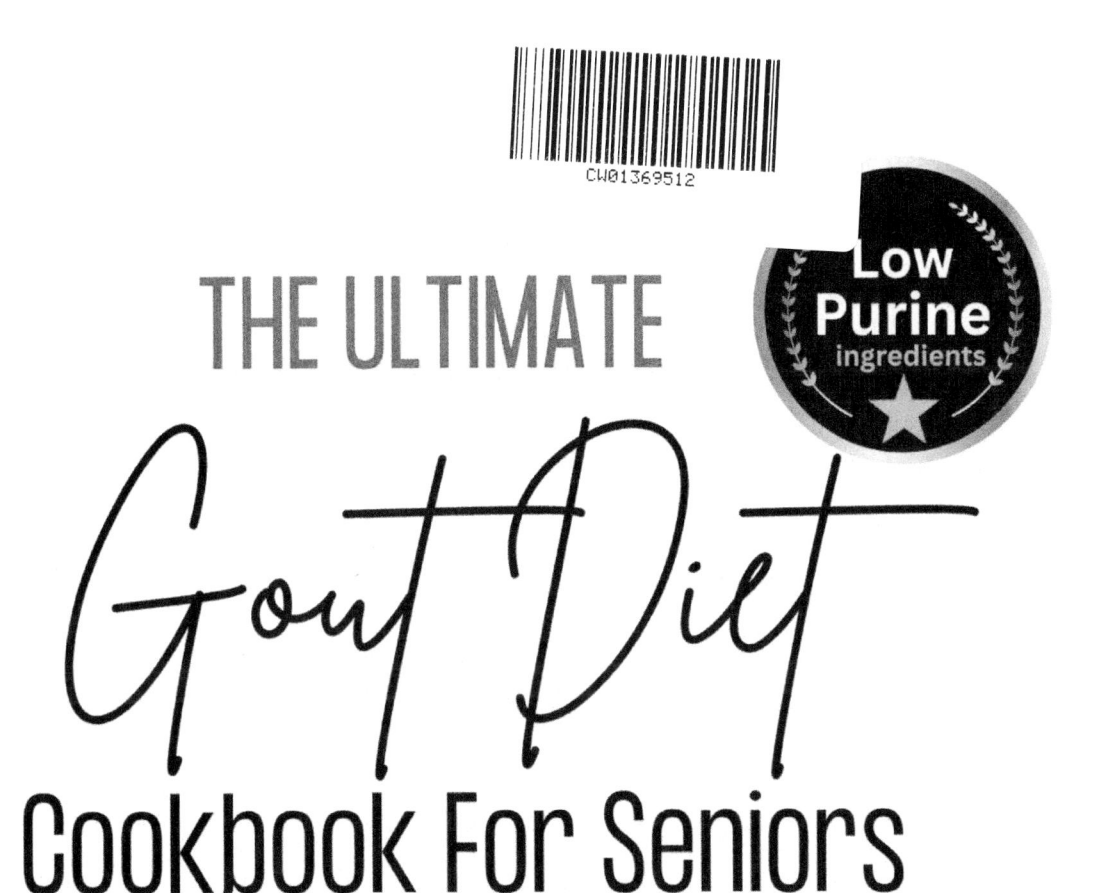

Simple and Delicious Low-Purine Recipes to Relieve Joint Pain, Reduce Uric Acid and Prevent Flare-Ups

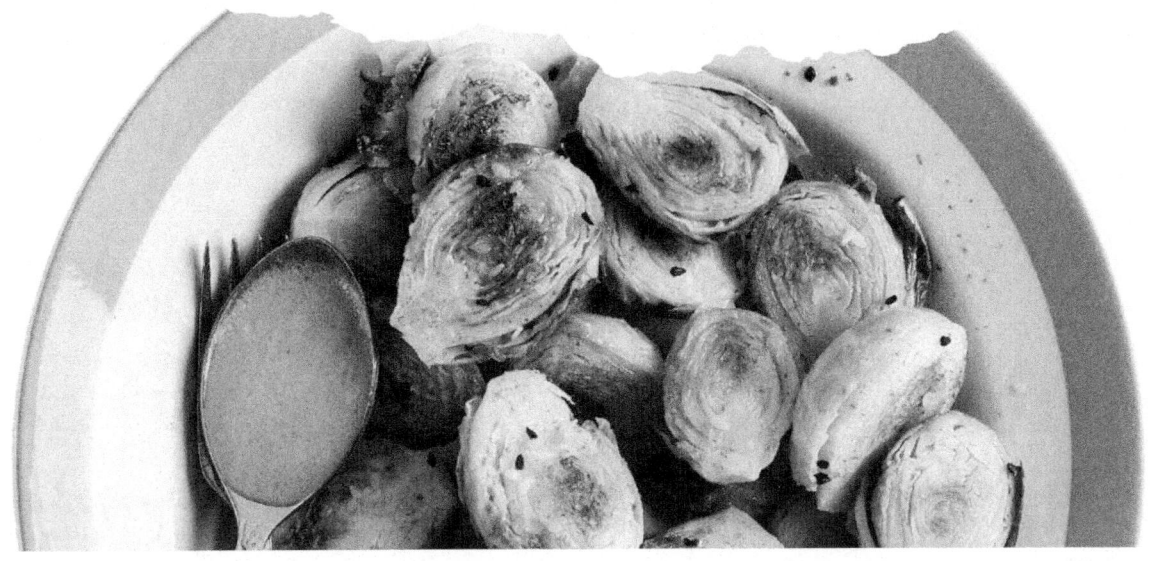

AMELIA SHARON

Copyright © 2025 by Amelia Sharon

All rights reserved.

No part of this publication may be reproduced, distributed, or transmitted in any form or by any means, including photocopying, recording, or other electronic or mechanical methods, without the prior written permission of the author, except in the case of brief quotations embodied in critical reviews and certain other noncommercial uses permitted by copyright law.

Disclaimer:

The content of this book is not intended to be a substitute for professional medical advice, diagnosis, or treatment. Always seek the advice of your physician or other qualified health providers with any questions you may have regarding a medical condition. Never disregard professional medical advice or delay in seeking it because of something you have read in this book.

TABLE OF CONTENT

INTRODUCTION 6

Welcome to a Pain-Free Life: How Diet Can Help Manage Gout 6

Understanding Gout: Causes, Symptoms, and Triggers 7

The Role of Diet in Managing Gout: What Science Says 8

What Are Purines? Understanding the Connection to Uric Acid 8

Why Seniors Are More Prone to Gout and How Diet Helps 9

CHAPTER 1: GOUT-FRIENDLY PANTRY ESSENTIALS 10

Must-Have Low-Purine Ingredients for Your Kitchen 10

What to Avoid: High-Purine Foods That Trigger Gout 12

Smart Grocery Shopping Tips for a Gout-Friendly Diet 12

Cooking Oils and Healthy Fats: What's Safe and What to Avoid 13

CHAPTER 2: 14

ENERGIZING BREAKFASTS FOR A PAIN-FREE MORNING 14

1. Carrot and Apple Oatmeal Bowl 14

2. Quinoa and Banana Breakfast Porridge 15

3. Almond Butter and Chia Toast on Whole-Grain Bread 16

4. Warm Cinnamon Quinoa with Berries 17

5. Scrambled Egg Whites with Roasted Vegetables 18

6. Coconut Yogurt with Chia and Flaxseeds 19

7. Sweet Potato and Avocado Breakfast Bowl 20

8. Zucchini and Goat Cheese Omelet 21

9. Turmeric-Spiced Golden Smoothie....21

10. Buckwheat Pancakes with Warm Berry Compote 22

11. Overnight Oats with Pear and Almonds 23

12. Pumpkin and Cinnamon Breakfast Muffins 24

13. Cucumber and Avocado Breakfast Wrap 25

14. Warm Lemon and Ginger Detox Tea 26

15. Spinach and Goat Cheese Scramble 27

16. Herbal Hibiscus Iced Tea 28

17. Papaya and Coconut Breakfast Shake 28
18. Flaxseed and Banana Energy Muffins 29

CHAPTER 3: LIGHT AND HEALING LUNCHES 30

1. Cucumber and Cottage Cheese Stuffed Peppers 30
2. Zucchini and Cucumber Salad with Lemon Dressing 31
3. Zucchini Noodles with Basil Almond Pesto 31
4. Chilled Cucumber and Yogurt Soup .. 32
5. Roasted Bell Pepper Hummus with Whole-Grain Pita 33
6. Baked Sweet Potato with Avocado Salsa 34
7. Green Goddess Quinoa Bowl 35
8. Broccoli and Almond Stir-Fry 36
9. Turmeric-Spiced Cauliflower Rice 37
10. Tomato and Herb Stew with Quinoa 38
11. Steamed Carrot and Green Pea Salad 38
12. Cabbage Slaw with Apple Cider Dressing 39
13. Zucchini and Goat Cheese Tart 40
14. Roasted Pumpkin and Kale Salad 41
15. Warm Beet and Walnut Salad 42
16. Baked Falafel with Cucumber-Tahini Sauce 43
17. Carrot and Ginger Soup 44
18. Butternut Squash and Apple Soup ... 44

CHAPTER 4: COMFORTING DINNERS FOR JOINT HEALTH 46

1. Herb-Roasted White Fish with Quinoa 46
2. Baked Lemon Chicken with Steamed Vegetables 47
3. Stuffed Bell Peppers with Brown Rice 48
4. Quinoa and Kale Stew 49
5. Grilled Eggplant with Garlic Yogurt Sauce 50
6. Roasted Zucchini and Quinoa Pilaf ... 51
7. Low-Purine Vegetable Stir-Fry with Brown Rice 52
8. Zucchini and Sweet Potato Casserole 53
9. Chickpea and Tomato Curry 54
10. Baked Cod with Lemon and Herbs .. 55
11. Butternut Squash and Kale Risotto .. 56
12. Pan-Seared Tofu with Sesame Greens 57
13. Roasted Brussels Sprouts and Almond Salad 58

14. Warm Beet and Goat Cheese Salad..60

15. Zucchini and Spinach Whole-Grain Pasta 61

16. Slow-Cooked Tomato and Quinoa Soup 62

17. Grilled Zucchini with Lemon Dressing 63

18. Sweet Potato and Carrot Mash.........64

CHAPTER 5: NOURISHING SOUPS & STEWS..65

1. Carrot and Ginger Soup 65

2. Butternut Squash and Apple Soup 66

3. Zucchini and Basil Soup 67

4. Creamy Cauliflower and Potato Soup 68

5. Slow-Cooked Tomato and Quinoa Stew 69

6. Sweet Potato and Carrot Soup 70

7. Pumpkin and Coconut Milk Soup......71

8. Broccoli and Almond Soup................72

9. Cabbage and White Bean Soup..........72

10. Mushroom-Free Vegetable Barley Soup 73

11. Zucchini and Leek Soup 74

12. Green Pea and Mint Soup 75

13. Spiced Apple and Carrot Soup.........76

14. Tomato and Red Pepper Soup..........77

15. Lemon Lentil Soup 77

16. Hearty Quinoa and Vegetable Stew .78

17. Kale and Sweet Potato Stew 79

18. Turmeric-Spiced Pumpkin Soup......80

CHAPTER 6: GOUT-FRIENDLY SALADS & SIDES....................................82

1. Cucumber and Avocado Salad with Lemon Dressing....................................82

2. Zucchini Noodles with Pesto 83

3. Carrot and Apple Slaw 84

4. Quinoa and Kale Salad with Citrus Dressing 85

5. Steamed Green Beans with Almonds.86

6. Roasted Sweet Potatoes with Garlic ..86

7. Pumpkin and Spinach Salad with Goat Cheese 87

8. Broccoli and Carrot Slaw...................88

9. Tomato and Bell Pepper Salad with Olive Oil..89

10. Steamed Brussels Sprouts with Lemon 90

11. Cauliflower Mash with Garlic..........91

12. Warm Beet and Walnut Salad...........92

13. Grilled Zucchini and Red Pepper Salad 93

14. Quinoa and Roasted Vegetable Medley 94

15. Carrot and Parsnip Mash.................95

16. Lettuce Wraps with Avocado and Chickpea Filling.......................96

17. Roasted Cabbage with Olive Oil......96

18. Butternut Squash and Kale Side Dish 97

CHAPTER 7: LOW-PURINE SNACKS & SMALL BITES..........................99

1. Baked Sweet Potato Fries 99

2. Carrot and Hummus Sticks 100

3. Cucumber and Avocado Roll-Ups ...100

4. Quinoa Crackers with Guacamole ...101

5. Almond Butter and Apple Slices......102

6. Steamed Edamame with Sea Salt.....103

7. Zucchini Chips with Paprika............103

8. Roasted Chickpeas with Turmeric ...104

9. Pumpkin Seed Trail Mix 105

10. Carrot and Ginger Energy Bites.....106

11. Frozen Banana and Almond Butter Bites 107

12. Coconut Yogurt with Chia Seeds ...107

13. Homemade Quinoa Granola Bars ..108

14. Baked Apple Chips with Cinnamon 109

15. Roasted Bell Peppers with Goat Cheese 110

16. Warm Pear Compote with Walnuts 111

17. Butternut Squash and Almond Smoothie 111

18. Herb-Roasted Kale Chips 112

CHAPTER 8: 28-DAY MEAL PLAN FOR GOUT RELIEF........................114

CONCLUSION 124

Lifestyle Tips Beyond Diet: Exercise, Hydration, and Stress Management 124

How to Handle Occasional Flare-Ups .125

INTRODUCTION

Welcome to a Pain-Free Life: How Diet Can Help Manage Gout

I remember the first time I saw my uncle struggle to walk. He was a strong man in his younger years always active, always on his feet. But as he got older, things changed. His feet would swell up overnight, and the pain would be unbearable. I can still hear him groaning as he tried to put on his shoes in the morning, wincing with every step. His hands, once so steady, began to show signs of stiffness. He was frustrated, not just by the pain but by the fact that something as simple as enjoying a meal could trigger such agony.

At first, he thought it was just aging, but then came the doctor's diagnosis **gout**. Like many seniors, he didn't fully understand what that meant at first. He just knew that certain foods made things worse. I remember watching him try to figure it out on his own, cutting out random foods, drinking more water, and hoping for the best. But nothing seemed to work.

That's when I started researching. I wanted to help him because I hated seeing him suffer. What I found shocked me **gout isn't just about aging. It's directly connected to what we eat.** The food choices we make every day can either **reduce pain and inflammation or trigger a full-blown flare-up.** When I helped my uncle change his diet, the difference was **life-changing.** The swelling reduced, the pain became manageable, and he could walk again without feeling like his joints were on fire.

If you're reading this, I imagine you (or a loved one) may be going through something similar. Maybe you've been told that gout is just something you have to live with, or that taking medication is the only solution. **But I'm here to tell you that food real, nourishing, low-purine food can be one of your greatest tools in managing gout.**

This book is designed to **guide you through simple and delicious low-purine meals** that will help **reduce uric acid buildup, ease joint pain, and restore your mobility.** No complicated recipes. No bland, restrictive diets. Just wholesome, satisfying meals that let you enjoy food without fear of another flare-up.

Understanding Gout: Causes, Symptoms, and Triggers

Gout is often misunderstood. Many people think it's just another type of arthritis, but in reality, it's much more than that. **Gout is caused by the buildup of uric acid in the blood, which forms sharp crystals in the joints.** Imagine tiny needles stabbing into your joints every time you move that's what a gout attack feels like.

It usually starts in the **big toe** a sudden, excruciating pain that wakes you up in the middle of the night. But it doesn't stop there. Gout can also affect the **ankles, knees, hands, wrists, and elbows.** Over time, if left unmanaged, it can cause **chronic pain, joint damage, and even kidney issues.**

The main triggers? **Diet.** Foods high in **purines** like red meat, organ meats, shellfish, alcohol, and sugary drinks cause the body to produce too much uric acid. If your body can't get rid of it fast enough, it crystallizes in the joints, leading to unbearable pain and swelling.

Many seniors struggle because they aren't aware of the connection between their **diet and their gout symptoms.** They continue eating high-purine foods without realizing they are fueling the very pain they want to get rid of.

The Role of Diet in Managing Gout: What Science Says

Scientific research has **proven** that dietary changes can **significantly** reduce gout attacks. Doctors recommend **a low-purine diet** because it helps lower uric acid levels naturally.

Here's what happens when you switch to a **gout-friendly diet**:

- Less inflammation – Your joints won't feel as swollen or stiff.
- Fewer flare-ups – No more waking up in the middle of the night in pain.
- Better mobility – You can move more freely without fearing the next attack.
- Improved kidney function – Your body will be able to eliminate uric acid more efficiently.

I've seen these benefits firsthand. My uncle, who once thought he'd have to live with constant pain, now enjoys life again. He can go on short walks, spend time in the garden, and even play with his grandkids without worrying about his feet swelling up.

This isn't just about avoiding pain it's about **taking back control of your life.**

What Are Purines? Understanding the Connection to Uric Acid

If you've never heard of **purines**, you're not alone. Many people don't realize that these natural compounds are in the foods we eat every day. When the body breaks down purines, it produces **uric acid.** Normally, your kidneys filter out the excess uric acid through urine.

But if you eat **too many purine-rich foods** or if your kidneys aren't eliminating uric acid properly (which is common in seniors), it starts to build up in your blood. **This is where the trouble begins.** The uric acid forms **sharp, needle-like crystals in the joints**, leading to swelling, redness, and intense pain.

That's why it's so important to choose **low-purine foods**, foods that don't overload your body with excess uric acid.

This book is filled with **delicious, satisfying meals that are naturally low in purines.** You won't have to guess what's safe to eat or feel deprived. Instead, you'll enjoy **nourishing, pain-relieving meals that let you feel in control again.**

Why Seniors Are More Prone to Gout and How Diet Helps

Gout isn't just a random condition it becomes **more common as we age** for a few key reasons:

✓ Slower kidney function – As we get older, our kidneys aren't as efficient at eliminating uric acid.
✓ Less muscle, more fat – Higher body fat can increase uric acid levels, while muscle loss can make mobility harder.
✓ Medications – Many seniors take medications for high blood pressure or other conditions that can interfere with uric acid removal.
✓ Dietary habits – Years of eating purine-rich foods without knowing their effects catch up with us over time.

But the good news is that **changing your diet can reverse a lot of these issues.** By eating **low-purine foods**, staying hydrated, and choosing **anti-inflammatory ingredients**, you can reduce symptoms and regain your quality of life.

The Ultimate Goal: Reduce Flare-Ups, Improve Mobility, and Enjoy Delicious Meals

At the end of the day, this book isn't just about recipes. It's about:

- **Living without constant fear of pain**
- **Enjoying food again without worrying about triggering an attack**
- **Being able to move freely and do the things you love**
- **Feeling empowered to take control of your health**

With the **right diet, the right ingredients, and the right recipes, you can enjoy food while keeping gout under control.**

I invite you to turn the page and start this journey with me. Let's cook delicious meals that **nourish your body, ease your pain, and give you back the life you deserve.**

CHAPTER 1: GOUT-FRIENDLY PANTRY ESSENTIALS

Managing gout through diet begins with **stocking your kitchen with the right ingredients**. The food choices you make daily can **either reduce inflammation and uric acid buildup or trigger painful flare-ups.** That's why it's essential to have a **gout-friendly pantry** filled with **low-purine, anti-inflammatory, and nutrient-rich foods** that support your health and mobility.

In this chapter, we'll explore:

✓ **Must-have low-purine ingredients** to keep in your kitchen

✓ **The best herbs and spices** for reducing inflammation

✓ **High-purine foods to avoid** that could trigger painful flare-ups

✓ **Smart grocery shopping tips** to help you choose the right foods

✓ **Safe cooking oils and healthy fats** for a balanced diet

By the end of this chapter, you'll be **fully equipped** to make **healthy, gout-friendly meals** without second-guessing your ingredients.

Must-Have Low-Purine Ingredients for Your Kitchen

The foundation of a **gout-friendly diet** is choosing **low-purine** foods that **won't contribute to excess uric acid buildup.** Here's a list of essential pantry staples that are **safe, nutritious, and delicious**:

1. Whole Grains

Instead of refined grains like white bread or sugary cereals, opt for **whole grains** that are **fiber-rich and low in purines**.

Examples include:

✓ Brown rice

✓ Quinoa

✓ Whole wheat pasta

✓ Oatmeal

✓ Barley

Whole grains help **stabilize blood sugar levels** and **support digestion**, which is essential for seniors managing gout. They also provide **long-lasting energy** without the uric acid spikes that refined grains can cause.

☞ Example: Instead of eating sugary breakfast cereals, try a warm bowl of

oatmeal with cinnamon and fresh berries for a fiber-rich, anti-inflammatory meal.

2. Low-Purine Protein Sources

Since red meat, organ meats, and shellfish are **high in purines**, it's important to replace them with **safe, low-purine proteins**

such as:

✓ Skinless poultry (chicken, turkey)

✓ Eggs

✓ Low-fat dairy (yogurt, cottage cheese, mozzarella)

✓ Plant-based proteins (tofu, lentils, chickpeas in moderation)

These protein sources **provide essential nutrients without the risk of uric acid buildup**.

👉 Example: Instead of a steak for dinner, prepare a **grilled chicken breast with steamed vegetables** a filling and gout-safe meal.

3. Fruits and Vegetables

Most fruits and vegetables are **low in purines and packed with vitamins, minerals, and antioxidants** that help reduce inflammation.

Some of the best options include:

✓ Cherries (known for lowering uric acid levels)

✓ Apples, pears, and bananas

✓ Berries (blueberries, strawberries, raspberries)

✓ Leafy greens (spinach, kale, Swiss chard)

✓ Cucumbers, bell peppers, and carrots

👉 Example: Instead of processed snacks, enjoy a refreshing **fruit salad with cherries, apples, and blueberries** to support your joints and overall health.

The Best Herbs, Spices, and Seasonings for Inflammation Control

Many seasonings can help **reduce inflammation and support joint health**. Instead of relying on **salt and artificial seasonings**, try these **gout-friendly herbs and spices**:

✓ **Turmeric** – Contains curcumin, a powerful anti-inflammatory compound that helps **reduce joint pain**.

✓ **Ginger** – A natural pain reliever that also **aids digestion** and boosts circulation.

✓ **Garlic** – Helps **lower uric acid levels** and fights inflammation.

✓ **Cinnamon** – Supports blood sugar control and adds a warm, rich flavor to meals.

✓ **Parsley** – A natural diuretic that helps the

kidneys **flush out excess uric acid**.

✓ **Basil** – Adds freshness to meals and has anti-inflammatory properties.

👉 Example: Instead of using high-sodium sauces, season your dishes with a mix of **turmeric, garlic, and black pepper** for an anti-inflammatory boost.

What to Avoid: High-Purine Foods That Trigger Gout

Certain foods are **major triggers for gout flare-ups** because they contain **high levels of purines**, leading to excessive uric acid buildup. Avoid these at all costs:

🚫 **Red Meat & Organ Meats** – Beef, lamb, pork, liver, kidneys, and heart are extremely high in purines.

🚫 **Shellfish & Seafood** – Shrimp, crab, lobster, sardines, anchovies, and tuna can spike uric acid levels.

🚫 **Alcohol** – Beer, liquor, and wine interfere with uric acid elimination.

🚫 **Sugary Drinks** – Soda and fruit juices with **high fructose corn syrup** can worsen gout symptoms.

🚫 **Processed & Fried Foods** – Chips, frozen meals, and fast food contribute to inflammation.

👉 Example: Instead of steak and beer, choose **grilled chicken with a cherry-infused herbal tea** both delicious and gout-friendly.

Smart Grocery Shopping Tips for a Gout-Friendly Diet

When grocery shopping, it's important to **make informed choices** to avoid high-purine foods and stock up on gout-friendly ingredients.

Here's how:

☑ **Shop the perimeter of the store** – Fresh produce, lean proteins, and dairy are usually on the outer aisles, while processed foods are in the center aisles.

☑ **Read labels carefully** – Avoid foods with **high fructose corn syrup, MSG, or artificial preservatives**, which can contribute to inflammation.

☑ **Buy fresh whenever possible** – Fresh fruits, vegetables, and proteins are better than canned or processed versions.

☑ **Plan your meals ahead** – Create a weekly meal plan to ensure you always have the right ingredients on hand.

👉 Example: Instead of grabbing frozen, pre-packaged meals, buy **fresh chicken,**

whole grains, and colorful vegetables for easy, homemade dishes.

Cooking Oils and Healthy Fats: What's Safe and What to Avoid

Not all fats are bad! Some fats **increase inflammation**, while others **help fight it**. Here's what to use and what to avoid:

✓ Safe, Gout-Friendly Cooking Oils:

- **Olive oil** – Rich in antioxidants and heart-healthy fats.
- **Avocado oil** – Great for cooking at high temperatures.
- **Flaxseed oil** – A good source of **omega-3 fatty acids**, which fight inflammation.
- **Coconut oil** (in moderation) – Contains healthy fats but should be used sparingly.

🚫 Oils to Avoid:

- **Vegetable oils** (corn, soybean, sunflower) – High in omega-6 fats, which can increase inflammation.
- **Margarine and shortening** – Contain **trans fats**, which worsen joint pain.
- **Processed butter substitutes** – Often contain additives that can trigger inflammation.

☞ **Example**: Instead of frying food in **vegetable oil**, use **extra virgin olive oil** for a healthier, anti-inflammatory choice.

Final Thoughts

Having the right ingredients in your kitchen is **the first step to managing gout through diet**. By replacing high-purine foods with **safe, low-purine alternatives**, you can reduce uric acid buildup, prevent flare-ups, and improve your overall well-being.

✓ **Stock up on whole grains, fresh fruits, vegetables, and lean proteins.**
✓ **Use herbs and spices that reduce inflammation.**
✓ **Avoid high-purine foods that trigger gout attacks.**
✓ **Choose healthy fats and oils to support joint health.**

With these essentials in place, you're ready to start cooking **delicious, gout-friendly meals** that help you live **pain-free and active!**

CHAPTER 2:
ENERGIZING BREAKFASTS FOR A PAIN-FREE MORNING

1. Carrot and Apple Oatmeal Bowl

Servings: 2

Prep Time: 5 minutes

Cook Time: 10 minutes

Total Time: 15 minutes

Nutrition Per Serving:

- Calories: 240
- Protein: 6g
- Carbohydrates: 42g
- Fiber: 7g
- Fat: 5g
- Sodium: 50mg

Ingredients:

- 1 cup rolled oats (low-purine whole grain)
- 2 cups almond milk (or low-fat dairy milk)
- 1 small apple, grated (anti-inflammatory and fiber-rich)
- ½ cup grated carrot (rich in beta-carotene)
- ½ teaspoon cinnamon (natural anti-inflammatory)
- 1 teaspoon chia seeds (high in omega-3s)
- 1 teaspoon honey (optional, for sweetness)
- ¼ teaspoon nutmeg (adds warmth and digestive benefits)
- 1 tablespoon chopped walnuts (optional, for crunch)

Instructions:

1. In a saucepan, heat the almond milk over medium heat until warm.
2. Add the oats and stir occasionally, cooking for about 5-7 minutes.
3. Stir in the grated apple, carrot, cinnamon, nutmeg, and chia seeds. Cook for another 2-3 minutes.
4. Once thickened, remove from heat and let sit for a minute.

5. Drizzle with honey (if using) and top with walnuts for extra texture.
6. Serve warm and enjoy!

Cooking Tips:

✓ Use **steel-cut oats** for a chewier texture.
✓ Swap **honey for maple syrup** if preferred.
✓ Add a splash of **vanilla extract** for more flavor.

Health Benefits:

✓ **Oats** – Low in purines, rich in fiber, and supports digestion.
✓ **Carrots** – Full of antioxidants and helps fight inflammation.
✓ **Apples** – Contain flavonoids that aid in **lowering uric acid levels**.
✓ **Chia seeds** – High in omega-3s, which help **reduce joint pain**.

2. Quinoa and Banana Breakfast Porridge

A protein-rich, low-purine, and anti-inflammatory alternative to traditional oatmeal.

Servings: 2

Prep Time: 5 minutes

Cook Time: 15 minutes

Total Time: 20 minutes

Nutrition Per Serving:

- Calories: 260
- Protein: 8g
- Carbohydrates: 45g
- Fiber: 6g
- Fat: 4g
- Sodium: 40mg

Ingredients:

- ½ cup quinoa (a great low-purine, high-protein grain)
- 1 cup almond milk (or oat milk)
- ½ cup water
- 1 small banana, mashed (provides natural sweetness)
- ½ teaspoon cinnamon (anti-inflammatory)

- 1 teaspoon flaxseeds (good for joint health)
- 1 teaspoon honey or maple syrup (optional)
- 1 tablespoon chopped almonds (for crunch, optional)

Instructions:

1. Rinse quinoa under cold water.
2. In a saucepan, combine quinoa, almond milk, and water. Bring to a boil.
3. Reduce heat, cover, and let simmer for 12–15 minutes until quinoa is soft.
4. Stir in mashed banana, cinnamon, and flaxseeds. Mix well.
5. Remove from heat and let it sit for 1-2 minutes.
6. Drizzle with honey (if using) and top with chopped almonds.
7. Serve warm and enjoy!

Cooking Tips:

✓ Use **coconut milk** for a richer texture.
✓ Add a pinch of **nutmeg** for extra warmth.

Health Benefits:

✓ **Quinoa** – Low in purines and rich in protein.

✓ **Banana** – Helps neutralize uric acid.
✓ **Flaxseeds** – Reduce inflammation and support joint health.

---

3. Almond Butter and Chia Toast on Whole-Grain Bread

A simple, protein-packed breakfast to keep you energized.

Servings: 2

Prep Time: 5 minutes

Cook Time: 0 minutes

Total Time: 5 minutes

Nutrition Per Serving:

- Calories: 280
- Protein: 9g
- Carbohydrates: 32g
- Fiber: 6g
- Fat: 12g
- Sodium: 120mg

Ingredients:

✓ 2 slices whole-grain bread (rich in fiber, helps digestion)

✓ 2 tablespoons almond butter (low-purine, high in healthy fats)

✓ 1 teaspoon chia seeds (anti-inflammatory)

✓ ½ teaspoon cinnamon (adds flavor and aids digestion)

✓ 1 teaspoon honey (optional)

Instructions:

1. Toast whole-grain bread until golden brown.
2. Spread almond butter evenly over the toast.
3. Sprinkle with chia seeds and cinnamon.
4. Drizzle honey for extra sweetness (optional).
5. Serve immediately.

Cooking Tips:

✓ Use **natural almond butter** without added sugar.

✓ Swap **whole-grain bread** for **sourdough** for easier digestion.

Health Benefits:

✓ **Almond Butter** – A good protein source that's gentle on the kidneys.

✓ **Chia Seeds** – Support joint lubrication.

✓ **Whole-Grain Bread** – High in fiber, promoting digestion and gut health.

4. Warm Cinnamon Quinoa with Berries

A nutrient-packed alternative to oatmeal, loaded with antioxidants.

Servings: 2

Prep Time: 5 minutes

Cook Time: 15 minutes

Total Time: 20 minutes

Nutrition Per Serving:

- Calories: 270
- Protein: 7g
- Carbohydrates: 46g
- Fiber: 8g
- Fat: 5g
- Sodium: 35mg

Ingredients:

✓ ½ cup quinoa

✓ 1 cup almond milk

✓ ½ teaspoon cinnamon

✓ 1 teaspoon vanilla extract

✓ ½ cup mixed berries (strawberries, blueberries, raspberries)

✓ 1 teaspoon flaxseeds

Instructions:

1. Cook quinoa in almond milk over medium heat for 12-15 minutes.
2. Stir in cinnamon and vanilla extract.
3. Add berries and let sit for 2 minutes.
4. Sprinkle with flaxseeds before serving.

Cooking Tips:

✓ Add **chopped nuts** for extra texture.
✓ Use **coconut milk** for a creamier version.

Health Benefits:

✓ **Berries** – Rich in antioxidants, help reduce inflammation.
✓ **Cinnamon** – Regulates blood sugar and fights inflammation.

5. Scrambled Egg Whites with Roasted Vegetables

A protein-rich, low-purine breakfast to keep you full and energized.

Servings: 2

Prep Time: 5 minutes

Cook Time: 10 minutes

Total Time: 15 minutes

Nutrition Per Serving:

- Calories: 220
- Protein: 14g
- Carbohydrates: 9g
- Fiber: 3g
- Fat: 10g
- Sodium: 180mg

Ingredients:

✓ 4 egg whites (low in purines and rich in protein)
✓ ½ cup cherry tomatoes, halved
✓ ½ cup zucchini, diced
✓ ½ cup spinach (use in moderation)
✓ 1 tablespoon olive oil
✓ ½ teaspoon black pepper
✓ ¼ teaspoon turmeric (anti-inflammatory)
✓ 1 teaspoon fresh parsley, chopped

Instructions:

1. Heat olive oil in a nonstick pan over medium heat.
2. Add cherry tomatoes and zucchini. Sauté for 3–4 minutes until tender.
3. Add spinach and cook for another minute until wilted.

4. In a bowl, whisk egg whites with turmeric and black pepper.
5. Pour the egg whites over the vegetables and scramble gently for 2–3 minutes.
6. Remove from heat and garnish with parsley.
7. Serve warm.

Cooking Tips:

✓ Cook on low heat to prevent overcooking.
✓ Add fresh basil for extra flavor.

Health Benefits:

✓ **Egg Whites** – High in protein, low in purines.
✓ **Tomatoes & Zucchini** – Rich in antioxidants.
✓ **Turmeric** – Reduces inflammation.

---

6. Coconut Yogurt with Chia and Flaxseeds

A gut-friendly, protein-packed, dairy-free breakfast.

Servings: 2

Prep Time: 5 minutes

Cook Time: 0 minutes

Total Time: 5 minutes

Nutrition Per Serving:

- Calories: 210
- Protein: 7g
- Carbohydrates: 20g
- Fiber: 6g
- Fat: 11g
- Sodium: 50mg

Ingredients:

✓ 1 cup unsweetened coconut yogurt (dairy-free, low-purine)
✓ 1 tablespoon chia seeds
✓ 1 teaspoon flaxseeds
✓ 1 teaspoon honey
✓ ¼ teaspoon cinnamon
✓ ½ cup fresh berries

Instructions:

1. In a bowl, mix coconut yogurt, chia seeds, flaxseeds, and honey.
2. Stir well and let sit for 5 minutes to thicken.
3. Sprinkle with cinnamon and top with fresh berries.
4. Serve chilled.

Cooking Tips:

✓ Add chopped nuts for crunch.

✓ Use almond yogurt as an alternative.

Health Benefits:

✓ **Chia & Flaxseeds** – Support digestion and joint health.

✓ **Coconut Yogurt** – Dairy-free, rich in probiotics.

---

7. Sweet Potato and Avocado Breakfast Bowl

A nourishing, fiber-rich breakfast with healthy fats.

Servings: 2

Prep Time: 10 minutes

Cook Time: 15 minutes

Total Time: 25 minutes

Nutrition Per Serving:

- Calories: 280
- Protein: 5g
- Carbohydrates: 40g
- Fiber: 7g
- Fat: 10g
- Sodium: 70mg

Ingredients:

✓ 1 medium sweet potato, diced

✓ 1 teaspoon olive oil

✓ ½ teaspoon paprika

✓ 1 small avocado, sliced

✓ 1 teaspoon chia seeds

Instructions:

1. Preheat oven to 375°F (190°C).
2. Toss diced sweet potatoes with olive oil and paprika.
3. Bake for 15 minutes or until tender.
4. Serve in a bowl with sliced avocado.
5. Sprinkle with chia seeds.

Cooking Tips:

✓ Add a poached egg for more protein.

✓ Serve with lemon juice for extra flavor.

Health Benefits:

✓ **Sweet Potatoes** – Anti-inflammatory, rich in fiber.

✓ **Avocado** – Provides healthy fats and potassium.

8. Zucchini and Goat Cheese Omelet

A light, protein-packed meal that's easy on digestion.

Servings: 2

Prep Time: 5 minutes

Cook Time: 10 minutes

Total Time: 15 minutes

Nutrition Per Serving:

- Calories: 230
- Protein: 12g
- Carbohydrates: 6g
- Fiber: 2g
- Fat: 15g
- Sodium: 120mg

Ingredients:

✓ 3 egg whites

✓ ¼ cup zucchini, grated

✓ 2 tablespoons goat cheese

✓ 1 teaspoon olive oil

✓ ½ teaspoon oregano

Instructions:

1. Heat olive oil in a nonstick pan.
2. Sauté grated zucchini for 2 minutes.
3. Pour whisked egg whites over the zucchini.
4. Cook for 3–4 minutes until set.
5. Add crumbled goat cheese and fold omelet.

Cooking Tips:

✓ Use **feta cheese** as a substitute.

✓ Add **fresh herbs** for extra flavor.

Health Benefits:

✓ **Egg Whites** – High in protein, low in purines.

✓ **Goat Cheese** – Easier to digest than cow's milk cheese.

---

9. Turmeric-Spiced Golden Smoothie

A soothing, anti-inflammatory smoothie packed with healing ingredients.

Servings: 2

Prep Time: 5 minutes

Cook Time: 0 minutes

Total Time: 5 minutes

Nutrition Per Serving:

- Calories: 180

- Protein: 5g
- Carbohydrates: 28g
- Fiber: 4g
- Fat: 6g
- Sodium: 40mg

Ingredients:

✓ 1 cup unsweetened almond milk

✓ ½ banana

✓ ½ cup mango chunks (fresh or frozen)

✓ ½ teaspoon turmeric powder

✓ ½ teaspoon ground cinnamon

✓ 1 teaspoon chia seeds

✓ ½ teaspoon honey (optional)

Instructions:

1. Add all ingredients to a blender.
2. Blend until smooth and creamy.
3. Pour into a glass and serve immediately.

Cooking Tips:

✓ Use frozen mango for a thicker texture.

✓ Add ginger for an extra anti-inflammatory boost.

Health Benefits:

✓ **Turmeric** – Reduces inflammation and supports joint health.

✓ **Mango & Banana** – Rich in vitamins and low in purines.

---

10. Buckwheat Pancakes with Warm Berry Compote

A gluten-free, fiber-rich breakfast to keep energy levels steady.

Servings: 4 (makes about 8 pancakes)

Prep Time: 10 minutes

Cook Time: 15 minutes

Total Time: 25 minutes

Nutrition Per Serving:

- Calories: 250
- Protein: 7g
- Carbohydrates: 45g
- Fiber: 5g
- Fat: 5g
- Sodium: 200mg

Ingredients:

✓ 1 cup buckwheat flour

✓ 1 teaspoon baking powder

- ✓ 1 cup unsweetened almond milk
- ✓ 1 tablespoon flaxseeds
- ✓ 1 teaspoon vanilla extract
- ✓ ½ teaspoon cinnamon
- ✓ 1 cup mixed berries (strawberries, blueberries, raspberries)
- ✓ 1 teaspoon honey

Instructions:

1. Mix buckwheat flour, baking powder, flaxseeds, cinnamon, and almond milk in a bowl.
2. Let the batter sit for 5 minutes to thicken.
3. Heat a nonstick pan and cook pancakes for 2–3 minutes per side.
4. In a separate pot, heat berries with honey for 5 minutes to create a compote.
5. Serve pancakes with warm berry compote.

Cooking Tips:

✓ Use a nonstick pan to avoid adding extra oil.
✓ Store extra pancakes in the fridge for 2 days.

Health Benefits:

✓ **Buckwheat** – Gluten-free and supports heart health.
✓ **Berries** – Antioxidant-rich and anti-inflammatory.

---

11. Overnight Oats with Pear and Almonds

A quick, make-ahead breakfast packed with fiber.

Servings: 2

Prep Time: 5 minutes

Cook Time: 0 minutes (overnight soak)

Total Time: 5 minutes + overnight soaking

Nutrition Per Serving:

- Calories: 220
- Protein: 6g
- Carbohydrates: 32g
- Fiber: 6g
- Fat: 8g
- Sodium: 50mg

Ingredients:

✓ 1 cup rolled oats

✓ 1 cup unsweetened almond milk

✓ ½ pear, diced

✓ 1 tablespoon sliced almonds

✓ ½ teaspoon cinnamon

✓ 1 teaspoon honey (optional)

Instructions:

1. Mix oats, almond milk, and cinnamon in a jar.
2. Add diced pear and almonds on top.
3. Refrigerate overnight.
4. Stir before serving.

Cooking Tips:

✓ Add a spoonful of chia seeds for extra fiber.

✓ Use steel-cut oats for a nuttier texture.

Health Benefits:

✓ **Oats** – Supports digestion and lowers cholesterol.

✓ **Pears** – Rich in fiber and low in purines.

12. Pumpkin and Cinnamon Breakfast Muffins

A warm, comforting breakfast that's gut-friendly.

Servings: 6 muffins

Prep Time: 10 minutes

Cook Time: 20 minutes

Total Time: 30 minutes

Nutrition Per Serving:

- Calories: 190
- Protein: 5g
- Carbohydrates: 28g
- Fiber: 4g
- Fat: 6g
- Sodium: 90mg

Ingredients:

✓ 1 cup oat flour

✓ ½ cup canned pumpkin

✓ 1 teaspoon cinnamon

✓ ½ teaspoon nutmeg

✓ 1 teaspoon baking powder

✓ 1 tablespoon flaxseeds

✓ ½ cup unsweetened almond milk

Instructions:

1. Preheat oven to 350°F (175°C).
2. Mix all ingredients in a bowl until combined.
3. Pour batter into muffin tins.
4. Bake for 20 minutes.
5. Let cool before serving.

Cooking Tips:

✓ Store in an airtight container for up to 3 days.
✓ Add walnuts for extra crunch.

Health Benefits:

✓ **Pumpkin** – Supports digestion and immune function.
✓ **Oat Flour** – Low in purines and gut-friendly.

---

13. Cucumber and Avocado Breakfast Wrap

A light and refreshing breakfast wrap packed with hydrating and anti-inflammatory ingredients.

Servings: 1

Prep Time: 5 minutes

Cook Time: 0 minutes

Total Time: 5 minutes

Nutrition Per Serving:

- **Calories:** 280
- **Protein:** 7g
- **Carbohydrates:** 34g
- **Fiber:** 9g
- **Fat:** 14g
- **Sodium:** 180mg

Ingredients:

✓ 1 whole-grain tortilla (or low-carb wrap)
✓ ½ avocado, mashed
✓ ½ small cucumber, thinly sliced
✓ ¼ cup alfalfa sprouts (or lettuce)
✓ 1 tablespoon Greek yogurt (optional)
✓ 1 teaspoon lemon juice
✓ ¼ teaspoon black pepper

Instructions:

1. Lay the tortilla flat on a clean surface.
2. Spread the mashed avocado evenly over the tortilla.
3. Layer cucumber slices and alfalfa sprouts on top.
4. Drizzle with lemon juice and sprinkle black pepper.

5. Roll the tortilla tightly and slice in half.
6. Serve immediately.

Cooking Tips:

✓ Use a **whole-grain or low-carb tortilla** for extra fiber.

✓ Add a dash of **turmeric powder** for added anti-inflammatory benefits.

✓ Keep the wrap fresh by wrapping it in parchment paper if taking it to-go.

Health Benefits:

✓ **Avocado** – Provides healthy fats that support joint health.

✓ **Cucumber** – Hydrating and anti-inflammatory.

✓ **Alfalfa Sprouts** – Rich in antioxidants and low in purines.

---

14. Warm Lemon and Ginger Detox Tea

A soothing, gut-friendly tea to reduce inflammation and support digestion.

Servings: 1

Prep Time: 5 minutes

Cook Time: 5 minutes

Total Time: 10 minutes

Nutrition Per Serving:

- **Calories:** 5
- **Protein:** 0g
- **Carbohydrates:** 2g
- **Fiber:** 0g
- **Fat:** 0g
- **Sodium:** 2mg

Ingredients:

✓ 1 cup hot water

✓ 1 teaspoon fresh ginger, grated

✓ ½ teaspoon lemon juice

✓ ½ teaspoon raw honey (optional)

Instructions:

1. Boil 1 cup of water.
2. Add grated ginger and let it steep for 5 minutes.
3. Strain into a cup and stir in lemon juice.
4. Add honey (if desired) and enjoy warm.

Cooking Tips:

✓ Use fresh ginger for the best anti-inflammatory benefits.

✓ Avoid honey if you prefer a completely sugar-free drink.

Health Benefits:

✓ **Ginger** – Reduces inflammation and aids digestion.

✓ **Lemon** – Helps alkalize the body and flush out toxins.

---

15. Spinach and Goat Cheese Scramble (Spinach in Moderation)

A light, protein-packed breakfast with just enough spinach to keep purine levels low.

Servings: 1

Prep Time: 5 minutes

Cook Time: 5 minutes

Total Time: 10 minutes

Nutrition Per Serving:

- **Calories:** 210
- **Protein:** 14g
- **Carbohydrates:** 4g
- **Fiber:** 1g
- **Fat:** 15g
- **Sodium:** 250mg

Ingredients:

✓ 2 egg whites (or 1 whole egg + 1 egg white)

✓ ¼ cup fresh spinach (moderate portion)

✓ 1 tablespoon goat cheese, crumbled

✓ 1 teaspoon olive oil

✓ ¼ teaspoon black pepper

Instructions:

1. Heat olive oil in a nonstick pan over medium heat.
2. Add spinach and cook for 1 minute until slightly wilted.
3. Whisk egg whites in a bowl, then pour into the pan.
4. Scramble gently for 2–3 minutes until cooked through.
5. Sprinkle with goat cheese and black pepper before serving.

Cooking Tips:

✓ Use **baby spinach** for a milder flavor.

✓ Stick to a **small portion of spinach** to avoid excess purines.

Health Benefits:

✓ **Egg whites** – Low in purines and high in protein.

16. Herbal Hibiscus Iced Tea

A refreshing, caffeine-free tea loaded with antioxidants.

Servings: 2

Prep Time: 5 minutes

Cook Time: 5 minutes

Total Time: 10 minutes

Nutrition Per Serving:

- **Calories:** 10
- **Protein:** 0g
- **Carbohydrates:** 2g
- **Fiber:** 0g
- **Fat:** 0g
- **Sodium:** 5mg

Ingredients:

✓ 2 hibiscus tea bags

✓ 2 cups water

✓ ½ teaspoon lemon juice

✓ Ice cubes

Instructions:

1. Boil water and steep hibiscus tea bags for 5 minutes.
2. Let the tea cool, then add lemon juice.
3. Serve over ice and enjoy!

Cooking Tips:

✓ Hibiscus tea is naturally tart, add honey if you prefer sweetness.

Health Benefits:

✓ **Hibiscus** – Supports blood pressure and uric acid balance.

---

17. Papaya and Coconut Breakfast Shake

A creamy tropical shake rich in digestion-friendly enzymes.

Servings: 1

Prep Time: 5 minutes

Cook Time: 0 minutes

Total Time: 5 minutes

Nutrition Per Serving:

- **Calories:** 200
- **Protein:** 5g
- **Carbohydrates:** 30g
- **Fiber:** 4g
- **Fat:** 7g
- **Sodium:** 50mg

Ingredients:

✓ ½ cup fresh papaya, diced

✓ ½ cup unsweetened coconut milk

✓ ½ banana

✓ 1 teaspoon flaxseeds

Instructions:

1. Blend all ingredients until smooth.
2. Pour into a glass and serve.

Cooking Tips:

✓ Use **ripe papaya** for natural sweetness.

Health Benefits:

✓ **Papaya** – Aids digestion and reduces uric acid buildup.

---

18. Flaxseed and Banana Energy Muffins

A fiber-rich, energy-boosting breakfast muffin.

Servings: 6 muffins

Prep Time: 10 minutes

Cook Time: 20 minutes

Total Time: 30 minutes

Nutrition Per Serving:

- **Calories:** 180
- **Protein:** 6g
- **Carbohydrates:** 30g
- **Fiber:** 5g
- **Fat:** 6g
- **Sodium:** 80mg

Ingredients:

✓ 1 cup oat flour

✓ 1 ripe banana, mashed

✓ 1 tablespoon flaxseeds

✓ ½ teaspoon cinnamon

✓ 1 teaspoon baking powder

✓ ½ cup unsweetened almond milk

Instructions:

1. Preheat oven to 350°F (175°C).
2. Mix ingredients until smooth.
3. Pour batter into muffin tins.
4. Bake for 20 minutes.
5. Let cool before serving.

Health Benefits:

✓ **Flaxseeds** – Rich in omega-3s and support digestion.

CHAPTER 3: LIGHT AND HEALING LUNCHES

1. Cucumber and Cottage Cheese Stuffed Peppers

A refreshing, protein-rich dish with anti-inflammatory benefits.

Servings: 2

Prep Time: 10 minutes

Cook Time: 0 minutes

Total Time: 10 minutes

Nutrition Per Serving:

- **Calories:** 180
- **Protein:** 10g
- **Carbohydrates:** 12g
- **Fiber:** 3g
- **Fat:** 8g
- **Sodium:** 220mg

Ingredients:

✓ 1 large bell pepper (red, yellow, or orange), halved and deseeded

✓ ½ cup low-fat cottage cheese

✓ ½ small cucumber, finely chopped

✓ 1 tablespoon fresh dill, chopped

✓ 1 teaspoon lemon juice

✓ ¼ teaspoon black pepper

Instructions:

1. In a bowl, mix cottage cheese, cucumber, dill, lemon juice, and black pepper.
2. Fill each bell pepper half with the mixture.
3. Serve immediately or chill for a refreshing meal.

Cooking Tips:

✓ Use **Greek yogurt instead of cottage cheese** if preferred.

✓ Chill for **30 minutes** before serving for extra flavor.

Health Benefits:

✓ **Cottage cheese** – High in protein but low in purines.

✓ **Cucumber** – Helps hydrate and flush excess uric acid.

2. Zucchini and Cucumber Salad with Lemon Dressing

A hydrating, crunchy salad packed with anti-inflammatory nutrients.

Servings: 2

Prep Time: 10 minutes

Cook Time: 0 minutes

Total Time: 10 minutes

Nutrition Per Serving:

- **Calories:** 120
- **Protein:** 3g
- **Carbohydrates:** 14g
- **Fiber:** 4g
- **Fat:** 6g
- **Sodium:** 50mg

Ingredients:

✓ 1 medium zucchini, spiralized or thinly sliced

✓ 1 small cucumber, thinly sliced

✓ 1 tablespoon fresh lemon juice

✓ 1 teaspoon olive oil

✓ ¼ teaspoon black pepper

✓ 1 teaspoon chopped fresh mint

Instructions:

1. In a large bowl, combine zucchini and cucumber slices.
2. Drizzle with lemon juice and olive oil.
3. Add black pepper and fresh mint.
4. Toss gently and serve chilled.

Cooking Tips:

✓ Let it **sit for 10 minutes** before serving for better flavor absorption.

✓ **Add avocado slices** for extra healthy fats.

Health Benefits:

✓ **Zucchini & cucumber** – Both are water-rich, reducing uric acid buildup.

✓ **Lemon juice** – Helps alkalize the body.

---

3. Zucchini Noodles with Basil Almond Pesto

A flavorful and nutritious alternative to pasta.

Servings: 2

Prep Time: 10 minutes

Cook Time: 5 minutes

Total Time: 15 minutes

Nutrition Per Serving:

- **Calories:** 250
- **Protein:** 6g
- **Carbohydrates:** 16g
- **Fiber:** 4g
- **Fat:** 18g
- **Sodium:** 120mg

Ingredients:

✓ 2 medium zucchinis, spiralized

✓ ¼ cup fresh basil leaves

✓ 2 tablespoons almonds, finely chopped

✓ 1 tablespoon olive oil

✓ 1 teaspoon lemon juice

✓ 1 clove garlic, minced

✓ ¼ teaspoon black pepper

Instructions:

1. Heat a pan over medium heat and lightly sauté zucchini noodles for **2-3 minutes**.
2. In a blender, combine basil, almonds, olive oil, lemon juice, garlic, and black pepper to create pesto.
3. Toss the zucchini noodles with the pesto and serve warm.

Cooking Tips:

✓ Don't overcook zucchini noodles—they should remain **slightly firm**.

✓ Store leftover pesto in the fridge for up to **3 days**.

Health Benefits:

✓ **Zucchini** – Low in purines and promotes hydration.

✓ **Almonds** – Provide anti-inflammatory healthy fats.

---

4. Chilled Cucumber and Yogurt Soup

A cooling, probiotic-rich soup perfect for soothing digestion.

Servings: 2

Prep Time: 10 minutes

Cook Time: 0 minutes

Total Time: 10 minutes

Nutrition Per Serving:

- **Calories:** 110
- **Protein:** 5g
- **Carbohydrates:** 10g
- **Fiber:** 2g

- **Fat:** 5g
- **Sodium:** 85mg

Ingredients:

✓ 1 small cucumber, peeled and diced

✓ ½ cup plain Greek yogurt

✓ 1 teaspoon lemon juice

✓ 1 teaspoon olive oil

✓ 1 teaspoon fresh dill, chopped

✓ ¼ teaspoon black pepper

Instructions:

1. Blend all ingredients until smooth.
2. Refrigerate for **30 minutes** before serving.

Cooking Tips:

✓ Serve **with a sprinkle of chia seeds** for added fiber.

Health Benefits:

✓ **Greek yogurt** – Rich in probiotics for gut health.
✓ **Cucumber** – Aids hydration and uric acid removal.

5. Roasted Bell Pepper Hummus with Whole-Grain Pita

A delicious, protein-packed spread with a smoky flavor.

Servings: 4

Prep Time: 10 minutes

Cook Time: 20 minutes

Total Time: 30 minutes

Nutrition Per Serving:

- **Calories:** 200
- **Protein:** 7g
- **Carbohydrates:** 28g
- **Fiber:** 6g
- **Fat:** 8g
- **Sodium:** 180mg

Ingredients:

✓ 1 large red bell pepper

✓ 1 cup cooked chickpeas (or low-purine alternative: white beans)

✓ 1 tablespoon tahini

✓ 1 tablespoon olive oil

✓ 1 teaspoon lemon juice

✓ ¼ teaspoon cumin

✓ ¼ teaspoon paprika

Instructions:

1. Roast the bell pepper in the oven at **400°F (200°C) for 20 minutes**, then peel and chop.
2. Blend all ingredients until smooth.
3. Serve with whole-grain pita.

Cooking Tips:

✓ Use **white beans instead of chickpeas** for a lower-purine option.
✓ **Roast the bell pepper** for deeper flavor.

Health Benefits:

✓ **Red bell pepper** – Rich in antioxidants and vitamin C.
✓ **Tahini** – Provides healthy fats for joint support.

---

6. Baked Sweet Potato with Avocado Salsa

A fiber-rich, anti-inflammatory dish packed with healthy fats.

Servings: 2

Prep Time: 10 minutes

Cook Time: 45 minutes

Total Time: 55 minutes

Nutrition Per Serving:

- **Calories:** 220
- **Protein:** 4g
- **Carbohydrates:** 38g
- **Fiber:** 8g
- **Fat:** 7g
- **Sodium:** 30mg

Ingredients:

✓ 1 large sweet potato, washed and halved
✓ 1 small avocado, diced
✓ ½ small cucumber, diced
✓ 1 teaspoon lemon juice
✓ ¼ teaspoon black pepper
✓ ½ teaspoon olive oil

Instructions:

1. Preheat oven to **375°F (190°C)**.
2. Place sweet potato halves on a baking sheet and bake for **45 minutes** until soft.
3. Meanwhile, combine avocado, cucumber, lemon juice, black pepper, and olive oil in a bowl.
4. Once sweet potatoes are done, top with avocado salsa and serve warm.

Cooking Tips:

✓ For **extra crunch**, sprinkle toasted pumpkin seeds on top.

✓ Bake **extra sweet potatoes** and store them for easy meals later.

Health Benefits:

✓ **Sweet potatoes** – Low in purines, high in fiber, and help with inflammation.

✓ **Avocado** – Provides healthy fats to support joint health.

---

7. Green Goddess Quinoa Bowl

A nutrient-dense, high-fiber dish that's perfect for lunch.

Servings: 2

Prep Time: 15 minutes

Cook Time: 15 minutes

Total Time: 30 minutes

Nutrition Per Serving:

- **Calories:** 260
- **Protein:** 9g
- **Carbohydrates:** 35g
- **Fiber:** 6g
- **Fat:** 10g
- **Sodium:** 80mg

Ingredients:

✓ ½ cup quinoa, rinsed

✓ 1 cup water

✓ ½ cup chopped spinach (moderate intake)

✓ ½ small cucumber, diced

✓ ½ avocado, diced

✓ 1 tablespoon olive oil

✓ 1 teaspoon lemon juice

✓ ¼ teaspoon black pepper

Instructions:

1. Cook quinoa in water for **15 minutes** until fluffy.
2. In a bowl, mix cooked quinoa, spinach, cucumber, and avocado.
3. Drizzle with olive oil, lemon juice, and black pepper. Toss and serve.

Cooking Tips:

✓ **Rinse quinoa well** before cooking to remove bitterness.

✓ Add a **sprinkle of hemp seeds** for extra nutrients.

Health Benefits:

✓ **Quinoa** – A low-purine grain, high in plant-based protein.

✓ **Spinach** – Anti-inflammatory (moderation recommended).

---

8. Broccoli and Almond Stir-Fry

A quick and healthy meal loaded with antioxidants.

Servings: 2

Prep Time: 10 minutes

Cook Time: 10 minutes

Total Time: 20 minutes

Nutrition Per Serving:

- **Calories:** 190
- **Protein:** 7g
- **Carbohydrates:** 15g
- **Fiber:** 5g
- **Fat:** 12g
- **Sodium:** 100mg

Ingredients:

✓ 1 cup broccoli florets

✓ 2 tablespoons sliced almonds

✓ 1 teaspoon olive oil

✓ 1 teaspoon lemon juice

✓ ¼ teaspoon black pepper

✓ 1 small garlic clove, minced

Instructions:

1. Heat olive oil in a pan over **medium heat**.
2. Add garlic and sauté for **1 minute**.
3. Add broccoli and stir-fry for **5 minutes** until tender.
4. Toss in almonds, lemon juice, and black pepper. Stir for **2 more minutes**.
5. Serve warm.

Cooking Tips:

✓ Use **light steaming** instead of stir-frying for a softer texture.

✓ For **extra protein**, add chickpeas (small portions).

Health Benefits:

✓ **Broccoli** – Rich in vitamin C, helps reduce uric acid.

✓ **Almonds** – Provide healthy fats for joint lubrication.

9. Turmeric-Spiced Cauliflower Rice *(Limited to ½ cup per serving)*

A light, anti-inflammatory alternative to regular rice.

Servings: 2

Prep Time: 10 minutes

Cook Time: 10 minutes

Total Time: 20 minutes

Nutrition Per Serving:

- **Calories:** 120
- **Protein:** 3g
- **Carbohydrates:** 15g
- **Fiber:** 4g
- **Fat:** 5g
- **Sodium:** 90mg

Ingredients:

✓ 2 cups cauliflower florets (processed into rice)

✓ ½ teaspoon turmeric powder

✓ ½ teaspoon olive oil

✓ ¼ teaspoon black pepper

✓ 1 small garlic clove, minced

✓ 1 teaspoon lemon juice

Instructions:

1. Pulse cauliflower florets in a food processor until rice-like texture forms.
2. Heat olive oil in a pan over **medium heat**.
3. Add garlic and cook for **30 seconds**.
4. Add cauliflower rice and turmeric, stir for **5 minutes**.
5. Season with black pepper and lemon juice, then serve warm.

Cooking Tips:

✓ **Don't overcook** cauliflower—it should be slightly firm.
✓ Pair it with **grilled vegetables or a light protein**.

Health Benefits:

✓ **Cauliflower** – Low in purines and packed with anti-inflammatory compounds.
✓ **Turmeric** – Contains curcumin, which reduces joint pain.

10. Tomato and Herb Stew with Quinoa

A comforting, fiber-rich stew that's easy on digestion.

Servings: 2

Prep Time: 10 minutes

Cook Time: 20 minutes

Total Time: 30 minutes

Nutrition Per Serving:

- **Calories:** 230
- **Protein:** 8g
- **Carbohydrates:** 32g
- **Fiber:** 7g
- **Fat:** 6g
- **Sodium:** 120mg

Ingredients:

✓ ½ cup quinoa, rinsed

✓ 1 cup water

✓ 1 medium tomato, diced

✓ ½ teaspoon dried oregano

✓ ½ teaspoon dried basil

✓ ½ small zucchini, chopped

✓ 1 teaspoon olive oil

Instructions:

1. Cook quinoa in water over **medium heat** for **15 minutes**.
2. In a separate pan, heat olive oil and sauté zucchini for **3 minutes**.
3. Add tomatoes, oregano, and basil, cooking for another **5 minutes**.
4. Mix in the cooked quinoa and serve warm.

Cooking Tips:

✓ **Rinse quinoa well** before cooking to remove bitterness.

✓ Add **a small handful of fresh parsley** for extra flavor.

Health Benefits:

✓ **Tomatoes** – Rich in antioxidants and vitamin C.

✓ **Quinoa** – A complete protein, perfect for a low-purine diet.

---

11. Steamed Carrot and Green Pea Salad

A simple, nutritious salad to keep inflammation at bay.

Servings: 2

Prep Time: 5 minutes

Cook Time: 10 minutes

Total Time: 15 minutes

Nutrition Per Serving:

- **Calories:** 140
- **Protein:** 5g
- **Carbohydrates:** 20g
- **Fiber:** 6g
- **Fat:** 3g
- **Sodium:** 50mg

Ingredients:

✓ 1 medium carrot, peeled and sliced

✓ ½ cup green peas

✓ 1 teaspoon lemon juice

✓ ¼ teaspoon black pepper

Instructions:

1. Steam carrots and peas for **10 minutes** until tender.
2. Transfer to a bowl, add lemon juice and black pepper.
3. Toss gently and serve.

Cooking Tips:

✓ Serve **chilled or warm**, depending on preference.

✓ Use **fresh peas** instead of canned for better taste.

Health Benefits:

✓ **Carrots** – Provide beta-carotene, which reduces inflammation.

✓ **Peas** – A moderate-purine food but fine in small portions.

---

12. Cabbage Slaw with Apple Cider Dressing

A crunchy, gut-friendly salad with a tangy twist.

Servings: 2

Prep Time: 10 minutes

Total Time: 10 minutes

Nutrition Per Serving:

- **Calories:** 110
- **Protein:** 2g
- **Carbohydrates:** 18g
- **Fiber:** 5g
- **Fat:** 4g
- **Sodium:** 20mg

Ingredients:

✓ 1 cup shredded cabbage

✓ ½ small carrot, grated

✓ 1 teaspoon apple cider vinegar

- ✓ ½ teaspoon olive oil
- ✓ ¼ teaspoon black pepper

Instructions:

1. Combine all ingredients in a bowl.
2. Toss well and let sit for **5 minutes** before serving.

Cooking Tips:

- ✓ **Massage cabbage** with vinegar for better texture.
- ✓ Add **a sprinkle of sunflower seeds** for crunch.

Health Benefits:

- ✓ **Cabbage** – Supports digestion and detoxifies the body.
- ✓ **Apple cider vinegar** – Helps with uric acid balance.

13. Zucchini and Goat Cheese Tart

A light, protein-packed tart perfect for a healing lunch.

Servings: 4

Prep Time: 15 minutes

Cook Time: 25 minutes

Total Time: 40 minutes

Nutrition Per Serving:

- **Calories:** 220
- **Protein:** 9g
- **Carbohydrates:** 22g
- **Fiber:** 3g
- **Fat:** 11g
- **Sodium:** 200mg

Ingredients:

- ✓ 1 small zucchini, thinly sliced
- ✓ ½ cup whole wheat flour
- ✓ 1 egg white
- ✓ ¼ cup goat cheese, crumbled
- ✓ 1 teaspoon olive oil
- ✓ ½ teaspoon dried thyme
- ✓ ¼ teaspoon black pepper

Instructions:

1. Preheat oven to **350°F (175°C)**.
2. In a bowl, mix **flour, egg white, and olive oil** until dough forms.
3. Press dough into a **lightly greased tart pan**.
4. Arrange zucchini slices over the dough and sprinkle with goat cheese.
5. Season with thyme and black pepper.

6. Bake for **25 minutes** or until crust is golden.
7. Let cool for **5 minutes** before slicing and serving.

Cooking Tips:

✓ **For extra flavor**, drizzle with a touch of honey after baking.

✓ If avoiding cheese, replace with a small amount of **mashed avocado**.

Health Benefits:

✓ **Zucchini** – Low in purines and packed with antioxidants.

✓ **Goat Cheese** – Lower in fat than cow's cheese and easier to digest.

---

14. Roasted Pumpkin and Kale Salad

A nutrient-dense salad packed with vitamins and minerals.

Servings: 2

Prep Time: 10 minutes

Cook Time: 20 minutes

Total Time: 30 minutes

Nutrition Per Serving:

- **Calories:** 180
- **Protein:** 5g
- **Carbohydrates:** 28g
- **Fiber:** 6g
- **Fat:** 5g
- **Sodium:** 40mg

Ingredients:

✓ 1 cup pumpkin, diced

✓ ½ cup kale, chopped

✓ 1 teaspoon olive oil

✓ ¼ teaspoon cinnamon

✓ 1 teaspoon lemon juice

Instructions:

1. Preheat oven to **375°F (190°C)**.
2. Toss pumpkin cubes with **olive oil and cinnamon**.
3. Spread on a baking tray and roast for **20 minutes**.
4. Let cool slightly, then mix with **chopped kale**.
5. Drizzle with lemon juice and serve.

Cooking Tips:

✓ **Massage the kale** with lemon juice to soften its texture.

✓ **Roast extra pumpkin** for use in soups or smoothies.

Health Benefits:

✓ **Pumpkin** – Anti-inflammatory and great for digestion.

✓ **Kale** – Contains antioxidants that help lower inflammation.

---

15. Warm Beet and Walnut Salad

A refreshing and hearty salad rich in anti-inflammatory compounds.

Servings: 2

Prep Time: 10 minutes

Cook Time: 20 minutes

Total Time: 30 minutes

Nutrition Per Serving:

- **Calories:** 200
- **Protein:** 6g
- **Carbohydrates:** 26g
- **Fiber:** 7g
- **Fat:** 9g
- **Sodium:** 35mg

Ingredients:

✓ 1 medium beet, peeled and diced

✓ ¼ cup walnuts, chopped

✓ 1 teaspoon olive oil

✓ 1 teaspoon balsamic vinegar

✓ ¼ teaspoon black pepper

Instructions:

1. Steam beets until tender (about **20 minutes**).
2. Let cool slightly and toss with **walnuts, olive oil, and balsamic vinegar**.
3. Season with black pepper and serve warm.

Cooking Tips:

✓ **For extra flavor**, sprinkle with **crumbled goat cheese**.

✓ **Use raw walnuts** instead of roasted to keep it heart-healthy.

Health Benefits:

✓ **Beets** – Help reduce inflammation and improve circulation.

✓ **Walnuts** – Contain omega-3s that support joint health.

16. Baked Falafel with Cucumber-Tahini Sauce

A light, protein-packed dish with a cooling sauce.

Servings: 2

Prep Time: 15 minutes

Cook Time: 20 minutes

Total Time: 35 minutes

Nutrition Per Serving:

- **Calories:** 250
- **Protein:** 10g
- **Carbohydrates:** 30g
- **Fiber:** 8g
- **Fat:** 9g
- **Sodium:** 120mg

Ingredients:

✓ ½ cup chickpeas, cooked and mashed

✓ ¼ teaspoon cumin

✓ ½ teaspoon garlic powder

✓ 1 teaspoon olive oil

✓ 1 small cucumber, grated

✓ 1 tablespoon tahini

✓ ½ teaspoon lemon juice

Instructions:

1. Preheat oven to **375°F (190°C)**.
2. Mix chickpeas with **cumin, garlic powder, and olive oil**.
3. Form into small patties and bake for **20 minutes**.
4. In a separate bowl, mix **cucumber, tahini, and lemon juice** for the sauce.
5. Serve falafel with the sauce.

Cooking Tips:

✓ Use **cooked chickpeas, not canned**, to reduce sodium intake.
✓ Serve in **a whole-wheat wrap** for a heartier meal.

Health Benefits:

✓ **Chickpeas** – A good source of protein and fiber without excess purines.
✓ **Cucumber** – Helps cool inflammation and hydrates the body.

17. Carrot and Ginger Soup

A warm, soothing soup that aids digestion.

Servings: 2

Prep Time: 10 minutes

Cook Time: 15 minutes

Total Time: 25 minutes

Nutrition Per Serving:

- **Calories:** 130
- **Protein:** 3g
- **Carbohydrates:** 22g
- **Fiber:** 5g
- **Fat:** 3g
- **Sodium:** 80mg

Ingredients:

✓ 1 cup carrots, chopped

✓ 1 teaspoon ginger, grated

✓ ½ teaspoon olive oil

✓ 1 cup vegetable broth

✓ ½ teaspoon black pepper

Instructions:

1. Heat olive oil in a pan and sauté ginger for **1 minute**.
2. Add **carrots and vegetable broth**, then simmer for **15 minutes**.
3. Blend until smooth and season with black pepper.

Cooking Tips:

✓ **Add a squeeze of fresh lemon** for extra flavor.

✓ Serve with **a slice of whole-grain toast**.

Health Benefits:

✓ **Ginger** – A natural anti-inflammatory for joint pain.

✓ **Carrots** – Support eye health and reduce oxidative stress.

---

18. Butternut Squash and Apple Soup

A naturally sweet, gut-friendly soup that is rich in fiber and anti-inflammatory nutrients.

Servings: 2

Prep Time: 10 minutes

Cook Time: 20 minutes

Total Time: 30 minutes

Nutrition Per Serving:

- Calories: 160
- Protein: 3g
- Carbohydrates: 34g
- Fiber: 6g

- Fat: 2g
- Sodium: 120mg

Ingredients:

✓ 1 ½ cups butternut squash, peeled and cubed

✓ 1 small apple, peeled and diced (Fuji or Honeycrisp work best)

✓ ½ teaspoon olive oil

✓ 1 cup low-sodium vegetable broth

✓ ½ teaspoon ground cinnamon

✓ ¼ teaspoon ground nutmeg

✓ ¼ teaspoon black pepper

✓ ½ teaspoon grated fresh ginger

✓ ½ cup unsweetened almond milk

Instructions:

1. Prepare the ingredients: Peel and cube the butternut squash and apple.
2. Sauté the aromatics: Heat olive oil in a pot over medium heat. Add grated ginger and cook for 1 minute until fragrant.
3. Simmer the vegetables: Add butternut squash, apple, vegetable broth, cinnamon, nutmeg, and black pepper. Stir well.
4. Bring to a gentle boil, then reduce heat and let it simmer for 20 minutes, or until the squash is tender.
5. Blend until smooth: Use an immersion blender to puree the soup until creamy. If using a regular blender, allow the soup to cool slightly before blending.
6. Add the final touch: Stir in almond milk for extra creaminess. Reheat for 1–2 minutes, if needed.
7. Serve warm, garnished with a sprinkle of cinnamon or a few pumpkin seeds.

Cooking Tips:

✓ For extra creaminess, use coconut milk instead of almond milk.

✓ Roast the butternut squash beforehand for a richer, caramelized flavor.

✓ Use a tart apple, like Granny Smith, if you prefer a slightly tangier taste.

Health Benefits:

✓ Butternut Squash – Low in purines, rich in vitamin A, and supports joint health.

✓ Apple – Provides fiber and antioxidants to reduce inflammation.

✓ **Ginger – A natural anti-inflammatory that aids digestion and joint pain relief.**

CHAPTER 4: COMFORTING DINNERS FOR JOINT HEALTH

1. Herb-Roasted White Fish with Quinoa

A light and protein-rich dish that supports muscle health while being low in purines.

Servings: 2

Prep Time: 10 minutes

Cook Time: 20 minutes

Total Time: 30 minutes

Nutrition Per Serving:

- **Calories:** 280
- **Protein:** 36g
- **Carbohydrates:** 28g
- **Fiber:** 4g
- **Fat:** 6g
- **Sodium:** 150mg

Ingredients:

- ✓ 2 fillets of white fish (cod, haddock, or tilapia)
- ✓ ½ cup cooked quinoa
- ✓ 1 tablespoon olive oil
- ✓ 1 teaspoon dried oregano
- ✓ ½ teaspoon garlic powder
- ✓ ½ teaspoon ground black pepper
- ✓ ½ teaspoon lemon zest
- ✓ 2 tablespoons fresh lemon juice
- ✓ 1 tablespoon chopped fresh parsley

Instructions:

1. **Preheat the oven** to **375°F (190°C)** and line a baking sheet with parchment paper.
2. **Prepare the fish:** In a small bowl, mix **olive oil, oregano, garlic powder, black pepper, and lemon zest.**
3. **Season the fish** on both sides with the mixture and place it on the baking sheet.
4. **Bake for 18–20 minutes** or until the fish flakes easily with a fork.
5. **Prepare the quinoa:** While the fish is baking, cook quinoa according to package instructions if not pre-cooked.
6. **Serve:** Plate the fish over a bed of quinoa, drizzle with fresh **lemon**

juice, and garnish with **chopped parsley**.

Cooking Tips:

✓ **Use fresh herbs** like thyme or rosemary for a more aromatic flavor.

✓ **Pair with steamed zucchini** or roasted carrots for a balanced meal.

Health Benefits:

✓ **White Fish** – A low-purine, high-protein source that's easy to digest.

✓ **Quinoa** – Rich in fiber and a great alternative to high-purine grains.

✓ **Lemon Juice** – Alkalizes the body and helps reduce inflammation.

---

2. Baked Lemon Chicken with Steamed Vegetables

A simple, nourishing meal that supports healthy joints while keeping purine intake low.

Servings: 2

Prep Time: 10 minutes

Cook Time: 25 minutes

Total Time: 35 minutes

Nutrition Per Serving:

- **Calories:** 320
- **Protein:** 38g
- **Carbohydrates:** 22g
- **Fiber:** 5g
- **Fat:** 7g
- **Sodium:** 160mg

Ingredients:

✓ 2 boneless, skinless chicken breasts

✓ 1 tablespoon olive oil

✓ 1 teaspoon dried basil

✓ ½ teaspoon garlic powder

✓ ½ teaspoon ground black pepper

✓ 1 tablespoon fresh lemon juice

✓ 1 cup steamed broccoli

✓ ½ cup steamed carrots

✓ ½ cup cooked brown rice

Instructions:

1. **Preheat oven** to **375°F (190°C)** and lightly grease a baking dish.

2. **Season the chicken:** In a bowl, mix **olive oil, basil, garlic powder, black pepper, and lemon juice**. Rub the mixture over the chicken breasts.

3. **Bake for 25 minutes** or until the chicken is cooked through (internal temperature should reach **165°F (74°C)**).

4. **Steam the vegetables:** While the chicken bakes, steam **broccoli and carrots** for **5–7 minutes** until tender.

5. **Serve:** Slice the baked chicken and plate it with **steamed vegetables and brown rice**.

Cooking Tips:

✓ **For extra moisture,** cover the chicken with foil while baking.

✓ **Use fresh herbs** like rosemary for a stronger flavor.

Health Benefits:

✓ **Chicken Breast** – A lean, low-purine protein option.

✓ **Broccoli & Carrots** – Anti-inflammatory and packed with vitamins.

✓ **Brown Rice** – Provides fiber and slow-releasing energy.

3. Stuffed Bell Peppers with Brown Rice

A nutrient-packed meal rich in fiber and antioxidants, perfect for a satisfying dinner.

Servings: 2

Prep Time: 10 minutes

Cook Time: 30 minutes

Total Time: 40 minutes

Nutrition Per Serving:

- **Calories:** 310
- **Protein:** 10g
- **Carbohydrates:** 48g
- **Fiber:** 8g
- **Fat:** 7g
- **Sodium:** 140mg

Ingredients:

✓ 2 large bell peppers (red or yellow)

✓ 1 cup cooked brown rice

✓ ½ cup diced zucchini

✓ ¼ cup diced carrots

✓ ¼ teaspoon black pepper

✓ ½ teaspoon dried thyme

✓ 1 teaspoon olive oil

✓ 1 tablespoon fresh parsley, chopped

Instructions:

1. Preheat the oven to 375°F (190°C).
2. Prepare the bell peppers: Cut off the tops, remove seeds, and lightly coat with olive oil.
3. Prepare the filling: In a bowl, mix cooked brown rice, diced zucchini, carrots, black pepper, and thyme.
4. Stuff the peppers: Fill each pepper with the rice mixture and place them in a baking dish.
5. Bake for 30 minutes or until the peppers are tender.
6. Garnish with fresh parsley and serve warm.

Cooking Tips:

✓ **For extra flavor,** add a teaspoon of lemon zest to the filling.
✓ **Use different colored bell peppers** for variety.

Health Benefits:

✓ **Bell Peppers** – Low in purines and rich in vitamin C, which supports collagen for joint health.
✓ **Brown Rice** – A whole grain that helps manage blood sugar levels.
✓ **Zucchini & Carrots** – Anti-inflammatory and easy to digest.

---

4. Quinoa and Kale Stew

A warm, comforting stew packed with anti-inflammatory nutrients to support joint health.

Servings: 2

Prep Time: 10 minutes

Cook Time: 25 minutes

Total Time: 35 minutes

Nutrition Per Serving:

- **Calories:** 290
- **Protein:** 12g
- **Carbohydrates:** 45g
- **Fiber:** 7g
- **Fat:** 6g
- **Sodium:** 160mg

Ingredients:

✓ ½ cup quinoa, rinsed
✓ 1½ cups vegetable broth (low sodium)
✓ 1 cup chopped kale (use in moderation)
✓ ½ cup diced carrots
✓ ½ cup diced zucchini

- ✓ ½ teaspoon dried oregano
- ✓ ½ teaspoon black pepper
- ✓ 1 tablespoon olive oil
- ✓ 1 teaspoon fresh lemon juice

Instructions:

1. In a pot, heat olive oil over medium heat.
2. Sauté carrots and zucchini for 3–4 minutes until slightly tender.
3. Add quinoa, oregano, and black pepper and stir well.
4. Pour in the vegetable broth, bring to a boil, then lower heat and simmer for 15 minutes.
5. Add chopped kale and cook for another 5 minutes until wilted.
6. Remove from heat, stir in lemon juice, and serve warm.

Cooking Tips:

✓ **Limit kale** to **1 cup per serving** as it contains moderate purines.
✓ **For extra protein,** add a handful of cooked chickpeas (in moderation).

Health Benefits:

✓ **Quinoa** – A low-purine, gluten-free grain high in fiber.

✓ **Kale & Carrots** – Rich in vitamins that reduce inflammation.
✓ **Olive Oil** – Supports heart health and reduces inflammation.

---

5. Grilled Eggplant with Garlic Yogurt Sauce

A flavorful, fiber-rich dish that helps fight inflammation and supports digestion.

Servings: 2

Prep Time: 10 minutes

Cook Time: 15 minutes

Total Time: 25 minutes

Nutrition Per Serving:

- **Calories:** 220
- **Protein:** 9g
- **Carbohydrates:** 24g
- **Fiber:** 8g
- **Fat:** 10g
- **Sodium:** 140mg

Ingredients:

✓ 1 medium eggplant, sliced into rounds
✓ 1 tablespoon olive oil
✓ ½ teaspoon ground black pepper

- ✓ ½ teaspoon dried basil
- ✓ ½ cup plain low-fat yogurt
- ✓ 1 clove garlic, minced
- ✓ 1 teaspoon lemon juice

Instructions:

1. Preheat a grill pan over medium heat.
2. Brush eggplant slices with olive oil and season with black pepper and basil.
3. Grill for 3–4 minutes per side until tender and lightly charred.
4. Make the sauce: In a small bowl, mix yogurt, minced garlic, and lemon juice.
5. Serve grilled eggplant with a dollop of garlic yogurt sauce.

Cooking Tips:

✓ **Use Greek yogurt** for a creamier texture.
✓ **Serve with quinoa or brown rice** for a complete meal.

Health Benefits:

✓ **Eggplant** – A low-purine vegetable that helps regulate blood sugar.
✓ **Yogurt** – Contains probiotics for gut health.
✓ **Garlic** – Anti-inflammatory and supports heart health.

---

6. Roasted Zucchini and Quinoa Pilaf

A nutrient-dense, high-fiber dish that makes a great light dinner.

Servings: 2

Prep Time: 10 minutes

Cook Time: 20 minutes

Total Time: 30 minutes

Nutrition Per Serving:

- **Calories:** 280
- **Protein:** 10g
- **Carbohydrates:** 44g
- **Fiber:** 6g
- **Fat:** 8g
- **Sodium:** 120mg

Ingredients:

✓ ½ cup quinoa, rinsed
✓ 1 cup low-sodium vegetable broth
✓ 1 medium zucchini, diced
✓ 1 tablespoon olive oil
✓ ½ teaspoon ground cumin

- ✓ ½ teaspoon black pepper
- ✓ 1 tablespoon chopped fresh parsley
- ✓ 1 teaspoon fresh lemon juice

Instructions:

1. Preheat oven to 400°F (200°C) and line a baking sheet with parchment paper.
2. Toss zucchini with olive oil, cumin, and black pepper, then roast for 15 minutes until golden.
3. Cook quinoa in vegetable broth for 15 minutes until fluffy.
4. Mix the roasted zucchini with quinoa and stir in fresh parsley and lemon juice.
5. Serve warm and enjoy.

Cooking Tips:

✓ **Roasting brings out the natural sweetness** of zucchini.

✓ **Pair with a lean protein** like grilled chicken or fish for a heartier meal.

Health Benefits:

✓ **Quinoa** – A high-fiber grain that helps regulate uric acid.

✓ **Zucchini** – Hydrating and rich in antioxidants.

✓ **Olive Oil** – Supports joint health.

---

7. Low-Purine Vegetable Stir-Fry with Brown Rice

A quick, nutritious stir-fry with anti-inflammatory vegetables to ease joint pain.

Servings: 2

Prep Time: 10 minutes

Cook Time: 15 minutes

Total Time: 25 minutes

Nutrition Per Serving:

- **Calories:** 320
- **Protein:** 9g
- **Carbohydrates:** 50g
- **Fiber:** 7g
- **Fat:** 8g
- **Sodium:** 180mg

Ingredients:

✓ 1 cup cooked brown rice

✓ ½ cup broccoli florets

✓ ½ cup sliced zucchini

✓ ½ cup chopped bell peppers (red or yellow)

- ✓ 1 small carrot, julienned
- ✓ 1 tablespoon olive oil
- ✓ 1 teaspoon low-sodium soy sauce
- ✓ ½ teaspoon turmeric
- ✓ ½ teaspoon garlic powder
- ✓ ½ teaspoon black pepper

Instructions:

1. Cook the brown rice according to package instructions and set aside.
2. Heat olive oil in a pan over medium heat.
3. Add broccoli, zucchini, bell peppers, and carrots to the pan and stir-fry for 5–7 minutes.
4. Add turmeric, garlic powder, black pepper, and soy sauce, then mix well.
5. Stir in the cooked rice and toss everything together for 2–3 minutes.
6. Serve warm and enjoy.

Cooking Tips:

✓ **Limit broccoli to ½ cup per serving** to keep purine intake low.
✓ **For extra protein,** add scrambled egg whites or pan-seared tofu.

Health Benefits:

✓ **Turmeric & Garlic** – Natural anti-inflammatories that help reduce joint pain.
✓ **Brown Rice** – A whole grain that supports digestion and energy levels.
✓ **Bell Peppers & Carrots** – Rich in vitamin C, which protects joints.

---

8. Zucchini and Sweet Potato Casserole

A satisfying, fiber-packed casserole perfect for a comforting dinner.

Servings: 2

Prep Time: 15 minutes

Cook Time: 30 minutes

Total Time: 45 minutes

Nutrition Per Serving:

- **Calories:** 350
- **Protein:** 11g
- **Carbohydrates:** 55g
- **Fiber:** 8g
- **Fat:** 10g
- **Sodium:** 160mg

Ingredients:

✓ 1 medium zucchini, sliced

✓ 1 medium sweet potato, sliced thinly

✓ ½ cup cooked quinoa

✓ ½ teaspoon dried thyme

✓ ½ teaspoon black pepper

✓ 1 tablespoon olive oil

✓ ¼ cup shredded low-fat cheese (optional)

Instructions:

1. Preheat oven to 375°F (190°C) and grease a baking dish.
2. Layer the zucchini and sweet potato slices in the dish, alternating them.
3. Sprinkle cooked quinoa between layers.
4. Drizzle with olive oil and season with thyme and black pepper.
5. Bake for 25 minutes, then add cheese on top (if using) and bake for another 5 minutes.
6. Serve warm and enjoy!

Cooking Tips:

✓ **Use thin slices** of sweet potato for even cooking.

✓ **For extra crunch,** top with crushed almonds or walnuts (in moderation).

Health Benefits:

✓ **Sweet Potato** – A low-purine, fiber-rich carb that helps digestion.

✓ **Zucchini** – Hydrating and loaded with antioxidants.

✓ **Quinoa** – A plant-based protein that helps with muscle and joint recovery.

---

9. Chickpea and Tomato Curry

(Chickpeas in moderation)

A mild, spiced curry that is both hearty and gentle on digestion.

Servings: 2

Prep Time: 10 minutes

Cook Time: 20 minutes

Total Time: 30 minutes

Nutrition Per Serving:

- **Calories:** 310
- **Protein:** 12g
- **Carbohydrates:** 45g
- **Fiber:** 9g
- **Fat:** 8g
- **Sodium:** 140mg

Ingredients:

✓ ½ cup canned chickpeas, rinsed and drained (use in moderation)

✓ 1 medium tomato, diced

✓ ½ cup chopped spinach (use in moderation)

✓ 1 teaspoon turmeric

✓ ½ teaspoon cumin

✓ ½ teaspoon black pepper

✓ 1 teaspoon olive oil

✓ ½ cup low-sodium vegetable broth

✓ 1 clove garlic, minced

Instructions:

1. Heat olive oil in a pan over medium heat.
2. Sauté garlic and diced tomato for 2–3 minutes until softened.
3. Add chickpeas, turmeric, cumin, and black pepper, then stir well.
4. Pour in vegetable broth and simmer for 10 minutes.
5. Stir in spinach and cook for another 2 minutes.
6. Serve warm, paired with brown rice or quinoa.

Cooking Tips:

✓ **Limit chickpeas to ½ cup per serving** to prevent excessive purine intake.

✓ **For a creamier texture,** blend half of the curry before serving.

Health Benefits:

✓ **Turmeric & Cumin** – Natural anti-inflammatory spices.

✓ **Chickpeas** – Provide plant-based protein but should be eaten in moderation.

✓ **Tomatoes** – High in antioxidants and vitamin C.

---

10. Baked Cod with Lemon and Herbs

A light, flavorful fish dish packed with anti-inflammatory benefits.

Servings: 2

Prep Time: 10 minutes

Cook Time: 20 minutes

Total Time: 30 minutes

Nutrition Per Serving:

- **Calories:** 280
- **Protein:** 34g
- **Carbohydrates:** 6g

- **Fiber:** 2g
- **Fat:** 12g
- **Sodium:** 120mg

Ingredients:

✓ 2 cod fillets (about 4 oz each)

✓ 1 tablespoon olive oil

✓ 1 teaspoon fresh lemon juice

✓ ½ teaspoon dried oregano

✓ ½ teaspoon dried thyme

✓ ½ teaspoon garlic powder

✓ ¼ teaspoon black pepper

✓ 1 small zucchini, sliced

✓ ½ cup cherry tomatoes, halved

Instructions:

1. Preheat oven to 375°F (190°C) and line a baking sheet with parchment paper.
2. Place cod fillets on the sheet and drizzle with olive oil and lemon juice.
3. Season with oregano, thyme, garlic powder, and black pepper.
4. Arrange zucchini slices and cherry tomatoes around the fish.
5. Bake for 18–20 minutes, or until fish flakes easily with a fork.
6. Serve warm, paired with quinoa or steamed vegetables.

Cooking Tips:

✓ **Use fresh cod** for the best texture and flavor.

✓ **Pair with brown rice or a side salad** for a complete meal.

Health Benefits:

✓ **Cod** – A lean, low-purine fish that supports heart and joint health.

✓ **Zucchini & Tomatoes** – High in vitamins and antioxidants.

✓ **Olive Oil** – A healthy fat that reduces inflammation.

---

11. Butternut Squash and Kale Risotto

A creamy, plant-based risotto rich in fiber and antioxidants.

Servings: 2

Prep Time: 10 minutes

Cook Time: 30 minutes

Total Time: 40 minutes

Nutrition Per Serving:

- **Calories:** 350

- **Protein:** 9g
- **Carbohydrates:** 55g
- **Fiber:** 7g
- **Fat:** 10g
- **Sodium:** 170mg

Ingredients:

✓ ½ cup Arborio rice

✓ 1 cup low-sodium vegetable broth

✓ ½ cup butternut squash, diced

✓ ½ cup chopped kale (in moderation)

✓ ½ teaspoon turmeric

✓ ½ teaspoon garlic powder

✓ ½ teaspoon black pepper

✓ 1 tablespoon olive oil

✓ 2 tablespoons grated Parmesan cheese (optional)

Instructions:

1. Heat olive oil in a pan over medium heat.
2. Add Arborio rice and stir for 1 minute to toast.
3. Gradually add vegetable broth, stirring frequently.
4. After 10 minutes, add diced butternut squash and continue cooking.
5. Once rice is soft (about 25 minutes), add kale, turmeric, garlic powder, and black pepper.
6. Stir in Parmesan cheese (if using), then serve warm.

Cooking Tips:

✓ **Stir frequently** to achieve a creamy texture.

✓ **Limit kale intake** to avoid excessive oxalates, which may affect some gout sufferers.

Health Benefits:

✓ **Butternut Squash** – Low in purines, high in fiber and vitamins.

✓ **Turmeric & Garlic** – Help reduce inflammation and joint pain.

✓ **Arborio Rice** – Provides energy while being gentle on digestion.

---

12. Pan-Seared Tofu with Sesame Greens

A protein-packed, plant-based dish with antioxidant-rich greens.

Servings: 2

Prep Time: 10 minutes

Cook Time: 15 minutes

Total Time: 25 minutes

Nutrition Per Serving:

- **Calories:** 320
- **Protein:** 18g
- **Carbohydrates:** 20g
- **Fiber:** 6g
- **Fat:** 18g
- **Sodium:** 190mg

Ingredients:

✓ 6 oz firm tofu, cubed
✓ 1 tablespoon olive oil
✓ ½ teaspoon black pepper
✓ ½ teaspoon garlic powder
✓ ½ teaspoon turmeric
✓ ½ teaspoon low-sodium soy sauce
✓ 1 cup baby bok choy, chopped
✓ ½ cup steamed green beans
✓ ½ teaspoon sesame seeds

Instructions:

1. **Press tofu for 10 minutes** to remove excess moisture, then cut into cubes.
2. **Heat olive oil in a pan** over medium heat.
3. **Add tofu cubes**, season with garlic powder, black pepper, and turmeric, and cook for **5–7 minutes** until golden brown.
4. **Add bok choy and green beans** to the pan, stir-frying for **3–4 minutes**.
5. **Drizzle with soy sauce** and sprinkle sesame seeds before serving.

Cooking Tips:

✓ **Use firm tofu** to keep its shape while cooking.
✓ **Steaming green beans** before stir-frying makes them more tender.

Health Benefits:

✓ **Tofu** – A great plant-based protein that is low in purines.
✓ **Bok Choy & Green Beans** – Provide fiber and essential vitamins.
✓ **Sesame Seeds** – Rich in healthy fats that help reduce inflammation.

---

13. Roasted Brussels Sprouts and Almond Salad (Limited to ½ cup per serving)

A delicious, fiber-rich salad with healthy fats for joint support.

Servings: 2

Prep Time: 10 minutes

Cook Time: 20 minutes

Total Time: 30 minutes

<u>Nutrition Per Serving:</u>

- **Calories:** 290
- **Protein:** 9g
- **Carbohydrates:** 26g
- **Fiber:** 7g
- **Fat:** 18g
- **Sodium:** 140mg

<u>Ingredients:</u>

✓ 1 cup Brussels sprouts, halved (limit to ½ cup per serving)

✓ 2 tablespoons almonds, sliced

✓ 1 tablespoon olive oil

✓ ½ teaspoon garlic powder

✓ ¼ teaspoon black pepper

✓ 1 teaspoon lemon juice

✓ ½ teaspoon honey

✓ ½ teaspoon Dijon mustard

<u>Instructions:</u>

1. Preheat oven to 375°F (190°C).
2. Toss Brussels sprouts in olive oil, garlic powder, and black pepper.
3. Spread on a baking sheet and roast for 15–20 minutes, flipping halfway through.
4. In a small bowl, mix lemon juice, honey, and Dijon mustard to make a dressing.
5. Toss the roasted Brussels sprouts with sliced almonds and drizzle with dressing.
6. Serve warm as a side or light dinner.

<u>Cooking Tips:</u>

✓ **Limit portion size** to ½ cup per serving to avoid excessive purines.

✓ **For extra crunch, toast the almonds** before adding them.

<u>Health Benefits:</u>

✓ **Brussels Sprouts** – High in fiber and antioxidants, but should be consumed in moderation.

✓ **Almonds** – Provide healthy fats and support joint health.

✓ **Olive Oil & Lemon Juice** – Help reduce inflammation.

14. Warm Beet and Goat Cheese Salad

A refreshing, antioxidant-rich dish that supports heart and joint health.

Servings: 2

Prep Time: 10 minutes

Cook Time: 30 minutes

Total Time: 40 minutes

Nutrition Per Serving:

- **Calories:** 260
- **Protein:** 7g
- **Carbohydrates:** 32g
- **Fiber:** 6g
- **Fat:** 12g
- **Sodium:** 130mg

Ingredients:

✓ 2 medium beets, roasted and sliced

✓ 2 tablespoons crumbled goat cheese

✓ 2 cups mixed greens (e.g., spinach, arugula, or romaine)

✓ 1 tablespoon olive oil

✓ 1 teaspoon balsamic vinegar

✓ ½ teaspoon Dijon mustard

✓ ¼ teaspoon black pepper

✓ 1 tablespoon chopped walnuts (optional, in moderation)

Instructions:

1. Preheat oven to 375°F (190°C).
2. Wrap beets in foil and roast for 30 minutes or until tender.
3. Let beets cool, then peel and slice into thin rounds.
4. In a small bowl, whisk olive oil, balsamic vinegar, Dijon mustard, and black pepper.
5. Arrange mixed greens on a plate, add sliced beets, and top with goat cheese.
6. Drizzle with dressing and sprinkle walnuts (if using) before serving.

Cooking Tips:

✓ **Roasting beets enhances their natural sweetness.**

✓ **If short on time, use pre-cooked beets.**

Health Benefits:

✓ **Beets** – Contain anti-inflammatory compounds that help with joint pain.

✓ **Goat Cheese** – Lower in lactose and easier to digest.

15. Zucchini and Spinach Whole-Grain Pasta (Spinach in moderation)

A comforting, nutrient-dense pasta dish perfect for a gout-friendly diet.

Servings: 2

Prep Time: 10 minutes

Cook Time: 20 minutes

Total Time: 30 minutes

Nutrition Per Serving:

- **Calories:** 340
- **Protein:** 12g
- **Carbohydrates:** 52g
- **Fiber:** 8g
- **Fat:** 10g
- **Sodium:** 150mg

Ingredients:

✓ 1½ cups whole-grain pasta (brown rice or quinoa-based)

✓ 1 small zucchini, spiralized or chopped

✓ ½ cup fresh spinach (limit to ¼ cup per serving)

✓ 1 tablespoon olive oil

✓ ½ teaspoon garlic powder

✓ ¼ teaspoon black pepper

✓ 1 teaspoon lemon zest

✓ 2 tablespoons grated Parmesan cheese (optional)

Instructions:

1. Cook whole-grain pasta according to package instructions.
2. In a pan, heat olive oil over medium heat.
3. Add zucchini and sauté for 5 minutes until soft.
4. Stir in spinach, garlic powder, and black pepper, cooking for another 2 minutes.
5. Drain pasta and mix with vegetables, tossing well.
6. Sprinkle with lemon zest and Parmesan cheese (if using) before serving.

Cooking Tips:

✓ **Use spinach in moderation** to prevent excessive purine intake.

✓ **For extra protein, add grilled chicken or tofu.**

Health Benefits:

✓ **Whole-Grain Pasta** – Provides fiber and supports digestive health.

✓ **Zucchini & Spinach** – Rich in vitamins and antioxidants.

✓ **Olive Oil & Lemon Zest** – Reduce inflammation and improve joint health.

---

16. Slow-Cooked Tomato and Quinoa Soup

A warm, hearty, and anti-inflammatory soup packed with fiber and plant-based protein.

Servings: 2

Prep Time: 10 minutes

Cook Time: 40 minutes

Total Time: 50 minutes

Nutrition Per Serving:

- **Calories:** 280
- **Protein:** 9g
- **Carbohydrates:** 45g
- **Fiber:** 8g
- **Fat:** 7g
- **Sodium:** 180mg

Ingredients:

✓ 1 cup cooked quinoa

✓ 2 medium tomatoes, chopped

✓ 1 small onion, diced

✓ 2 cups low-sodium vegetable broth

✓ 1 teaspoon olive oil

✓ ½ teaspoon garlic powder

✓ ½ teaspoon turmeric

✓ ¼ teaspoon black pepper

✓ ½ teaspoon dried basil

Instructions:

1. Heat olive oil in a pot over medium heat.
2. Sauté onions for 3–4 minutes until soft.
3. Add chopped tomatoes, garlic powder, turmeric, and black pepper.
4. Pour in vegetable broth and bring to a simmer.
5. Let it cook for 30 minutes, stirring occasionally.
6. Add cooked quinoa and dried basil, stirring well.
7. Simmer for another 5 minutes, then serve warm.

Cooking Tips:

✓ For a smoother texture, blend the soup before adding quinoa.

✓ Top with a squeeze of lemon juice for added freshness.

Health Benefits:

✓ **Tomatoes** – Rich in antioxidants like lycopene, which fights inflammation.

✓ **Quinoa** – A high-fiber, low-purine grain that helps digestion.

✓ **Turmeric** – Contains curcumin, which reduces joint pain.

17. Grilled Zucchini with Lemon Dressing

A light and flavorful dish loaded with anti-inflammatory benefits.

Servings: 2

Prep Time: 5 minutes

Cook Time: 10 minutes

Total Time: 15 minutes

Nutrition Per Serving:

- **Calories:** 160
- **Protein:** 4g
- **Carbohydrates:** 12g
- **Fiber:** 4g
- **Fat:** 10g
- **Sodium:** 120mg

Ingredients:

✓ 2 medium zucchinis, sliced lengthwise

✓ 1 tablespoon olive oil

✓ ½ teaspoon garlic powder

✓ ¼ teaspoon black pepper

✓ 1 teaspoon lemon juice

✓ 1 teaspoon chopped parsley

Instructions:

1. Preheat grill or stovetop grill pan over medium heat.
2. Brush zucchini slices with olive oil and sprinkle garlic powder and black pepper.
3. Grill for about 3–4 minutes per side until soft and slightly charred.
4. Transfer to a plate and drizzle with lemon juice.
5. Sprinkle chopped parsley before serving.

Cooking Tips:

✓ For extra flavor, marinate zucchini for 15 minutes before grilling.

✓ Serve as a side dish or mix with quinoa for a full meal.

Health Benefits:

✓ **Zucchini** – Low in purines and high in antioxidants.

✓ **Olive Oil & Lemon Juice** – Help reduce inflammation and aid digestion.

✓ **Garlic & Parsley** – Support immune health and provide anti-inflammatory properties.

---

18. Sweet Potato and Carrot Mash

A naturally sweet, nutrient-packed side dish to complement any meal.

Servings: 2

Prep Time: 10 minutes

Cook Time: 25 minutes

Total Time: 35 minutes

Nutrition Per Serving:

- **Calories:** 230
- **Protein:** 3g
- **Carbohydrates:** 45g
- **Fiber:** 7g
- **Fat:** 6g
- **Sodium:** 100mg

Ingredients:

✓ 1 medium sweet potato, peeled and chopped

✓ 2 medium carrots, peeled and chopped

✓ 1 tablespoon olive oil

✓ ½ teaspoon cinnamon

✓ ¼ teaspoon nutmeg

✓ ¼ teaspoon black pepper

✓ 2 tablespoons unsweetened almond milk

Instructions:

1. Boil sweet potatoes and carrots in a pot of water for 20 minutes until tender.
2. Drain and transfer to a mixing bowl.
3. Mash well with a fork or potato masher.
4. Add olive oil, almond milk, cinnamon, nutmeg, and black pepper.
5. Mix until smooth and creamy, then serve warm.

Cooking Tips:

✓ For extra creaminess, use a hand blender.

✓ Pairs well with baked fish or grilled chicken.

CHAPTER 5: NOURISHING SOUPS & STEWS

1. Carrot and Ginger Soup

A warming, anti-inflammatory soup packed with beta-carotene and digestion-boosting ginger.

Servings: 2

Prep Time: 10 minutes

Cook Time: 20 minutes

Total Time: 30 minutes

Nutrition Per Serving:

- **Calories:** 180
- **Protein:** 3g
- **Carbohydrates:** 35g
- **Fiber:** 6g
- **Fat:** 5g
- **Sodium:** 140mg

Ingredients:

✓ 2 large carrots, peeled and chopped

✓ ½ small onion, diced

✓ 1 teaspoon grated fresh ginger

✓ 2 cups low-sodium vegetable broth

✓ 1 teaspoon olive oil

✓ ½ teaspoon turmeric

✓ ¼ teaspoon black pepper

✓ ¼ teaspoon cumin

✓ 1 tablespoon lemon juice

Instructions:

1. Heat olive oil in a pot over medium heat.
2. Sauté onions for 3–4 minutes until translucent.
3. Add carrots, ginger, turmeric, cumin, and black pepper. Stir well.
4. Pour in vegetable broth and bring to a boil. Reduce heat and simmer for 15 minutes until carrots are soft.
5. Blend the soup using an immersion blender until smooth.
6. Stir in lemon juice and serve warm.

Cooking Tips:

✓ For a creamier texture, add 2 tablespoons of unsweetened almond milk.

✓ Garnish with chopped parsley or a drizzle of olive oil.

Health Benefits:

✓ **Carrots** – Rich in beta-carotene, which reduces inflammation.

✓ **Ginger & Turmeric** – Help reduce joint pain and boost digestion.

✓ **Lemon Juice** – Aids detoxification and supports kidney health.

---

2. Butternut Squash and Apple Soup

A naturally sweet, gut-friendly soup rich in antioxidants.

Servings: 2

Prep Time: 10 minutes

Cook Time: 20 minutes

Total Time: 30 minutes

Nutrition Per Serving:

- **Calories:** 220
- **Protein:** 3g
- **Carbohydrates:** 45g
- **Fiber:** 7g
- **Fat:** 5g
- **Sodium:** 160mg

Ingredients:

✓ 1 cup diced butternut squash

✓ 1 small apple, peeled and chopped

✓ ½ small onion, diced

✓ 2 cups low-sodium vegetable broth

✓ 1 teaspoon olive oil

✓ ½ teaspoon cinnamon

✓ ¼ teaspoon nutmeg

✓ ¼ teaspoon black pepper

Instructions:

1. Heat olive oil in a pot over medium heat.
2. Sauté onions for 3–4 minutes until soft.
3. Add butternut squash, apple, cinnamon, nutmeg, and black pepper. Stir well.
4. Pour in vegetable broth and bring to a boil. Reduce heat and simmer for 20 minutes.
5. Blend the soup until smooth and serve warm.

Cooking Tips:

✓ For extra creaminess, stir in 1 tablespoon of coconut milk.

✓ Garnish with toasted pumpkin seeds for crunch.

Health Benefits:

✓ **Butternut Squash & Apple** – High in fiber and antioxidants.

✓ **Cinnamon & Nutmeg** – Help regulate blood sugar and inflammation.

✓ **Olive Oil** – Provides healthy fats that support joint health.

---

3. Zucchini and Basil Soup

A light, refreshing, and anti-inflammatory soup perfect for digestion.

Servings: 2

Prep Time: 10 minutes

Cook Time: 15 minutes

Total Time: 25 minutes

Nutrition Per Serving:

- **Calories:** 140
- **Protein:** 4g
- **Carbohydrates:** 18g
- **Fiber:** 5g
- **Fat:** 6g
- **Sodium:** 110mg

Ingredients:

✓ 1 medium zucchini, chopped

✓ ½ small onion, diced

✓ 1 cup fresh basil leaves

✓ 2 cups low-sodium vegetable broth

✓ 1 teaspoon olive oil

✓ ¼ teaspoon garlic powder

✓ ¼ teaspoon black pepper

Instructions:

1. Heat olive oil in a pot over medium heat.
2. Sauté onions for 3–4 minutes until soft.
3. Add zucchini, garlic powder, and black pepper. Stir well.
4. Pour in vegetable broth and simmer for 10 minutes.
5. Blend the soup until smooth.
6. Stir in fresh basil before serving.

Cooking Tips:

✓ For a creamy version, add 2 tablespoons of coconut yogurt.

✓ Garnish with chopped almonds for texture.

Health Benefits:

✓ **Zucchini** – Low in purines and supports digestion.
✓ **Basil** – Contains anti-inflammatory compounds that reduce joint pain.

---

4. Creamy Cauliflower and Potato Soup (Limit cauliflower to ½ cup per serving)

A hearty, low-purine alternative to traditional creamy soups.

Servings: 2

Prep Time: 10 minutes

Cook Time: 25 minutes

Total Time: 35 minutes

Nutrition Per Serving:

- **Calories:** 190
- **Protein:** 5g
- **Carbohydrates:** 32g
- **Fiber:** 6g
- **Fat:** 5g
- **Sodium:** 140mg

Ingredients:

✓ ½ cup chopped cauliflower
✓ 1 medium potato, diced
✓ ½ small onion, diced
✓ 2 cups low-sodium vegetable broth
✓ 1 teaspoon olive oil
✓ ½ teaspoon thyme
✓ ¼ teaspoon black pepper

Instructions:

1. Heat olive oil in a pot over medium heat.
2. Sauté onions for 3–4 minutes until soft.
3. Add cauliflower, potato, thyme, and black pepper. Stir well.
4. Pour in vegetable broth and simmer for 25 minutes.
5. Blend the soup until smooth and creamy.

Health Benefits:

✓ **Cauliflower & Potato** – Provide fiber and antioxidants.
✓ **Thyme & Black Pepper** – Support digestion and reduce inflammation.

5. Slow-Cooked Tomato and Quinoa Stew

A hearty, fiber-rich stew that's low in purines and packed with anti-inflammatory ingredients.

Servings: 2

Prep Time: 10 minutes

Cook Time: 35 minutes

Total Time: 45 minutes

Nutrition Per Serving:

- **Calories:** 210
- **Protein:** 7g
- **Carbohydrates:** 38g
- **Fiber:** 8g
- **Fat:** 4g
- **Sodium:** 160mg

Ingredients:

✓ 1 cup diced tomatoes (fresh or canned, no added salt)
✓ ½ cup cooked quinoa
✓ ½ small onion, diced
✓ 1 carrot, diced
✓ 1 celery stalk, chopped
✓ 2 cups low-sodium vegetable broth
✓ 1 teaspoon olive oil
✓ ½ teaspoon cumin
✓ ¼ teaspoon black pepper
✓ ½ teaspoon dried oregano

Instructions:

1. Heat olive oil in a pot over medium heat.
2. Sauté onions, carrots, and celery for 5 minutes until soft.
3. Add diced tomatoes, quinoa, cumin, black pepper, and oregano. Stir well.
4. Pour in vegetable broth and bring to a boil.
5. Reduce heat and simmer for 30 minutes, stirring occasionally.
6. Serve warm, garnished with fresh parsley.

Cooking Tips:

✓ For a thicker consistency, mash some of the tomatoes while cooking.
✓ You can replace quinoa with brown rice for variety.

Health Benefits:

✓ **Quinoa** – Low in purines and rich in fiber.

6. Sweet Potato and Carrot Soup

A naturally sweet, vitamin-rich soup that's easy to digest and gentle on joints.

Servings: 2

Prep Time: 10 minutes

Cook Time: 20 minutes

Total Time: 30 minutes

Nutrition Per Serving:

- **Calories:** 200
- **Protein:** 4g
- **Carbohydrates:** 40g
- **Fiber:** 7g
- **Fat:** 3g
- **Sodium:** 140mg

Ingredients:

✓ 1 medium sweet potato, peeled and diced

✓ 1 large carrot, chopped

✓ ½ small onion, diced

✓ 2 cups low-sodium vegetable broth

✓ 1 teaspoon olive oil

✓ ½ teaspoon turmeric

✓ ¼ teaspoon black pepper

✓ ½ teaspoon cinnamon

Instructions:

1. Heat olive oil in a pot over medium heat.
2. Sauté onions for 3 minutes until soft.
3. Add sweet potato, carrot, turmeric, black pepper, and cinnamon. Stir well.
4. Pour in vegetable broth and bring to a boil.
5. Reduce heat and simmer for 20 minutes.
6. Blend the soup until smooth and creamy.

Cooking Tips:

✓ Add a dash of coconut milk for extra creaminess.

✓ Garnish with pumpkin seeds for texture.

Health Benefits:

✓ **Sweet Potatoes & Carrots** – High in antioxidants and fiber.

✓ **Turmeric & Cinnamon** – Help reduce joint inflammation.

7. Pumpkin and Coconut Milk Soup

A creamy, immune-boosting soup that's rich in anti-inflammatory nutrients.

Servings: 2

Prep Time: 10 minutes

Cook Time: 25 minutes

Total Time: 35 minutes

Nutrition Per Serving:

- **Calories:** 220
- **Protein:** 3g
- **Carbohydrates:** 35g
- **Fiber:** 5g
- **Fat:** 8g
- **Sodium:** 130mg

Ingredients:

✓ 1 cup pumpkin purée (or cooked fresh pumpkin)
✓ 1 cup unsweetened coconut milk
✓ 1 cup low-sodium vegetable broth
✓ ½ small onion, diced
✓ ½ teaspoon turmeric
✓ ¼ teaspoon black pepper
✓ ½ teaspoon ginger powder

Instructions:

1. **Heat a pot over medium heat and sauté onions for 3 minutes.**
2. **Add pumpkin purée, coconut milk, turmeric, black pepper, and ginger powder.** Stir well.
3. **Pour in vegetable broth and bring to a simmer.**
4. **Cook for 20 minutes, stirring occasionally.**
5. **Blend for a smooth texture and serve warm.**

Cooking Tips:

✓ Top with roasted pumpkin seeds for a crunchy contrast.
✓ A drizzle of lemon juice enhances the flavor.

Health Benefits:

✓ **Pumpkin** – High in beta-carotene for immune and joint health.
✓ **Coconut Milk** – Provides healthy fats for joint lubrication.

8. Broccoli and Almond Soup

A light and nutritious soup with a touch of nutty flavor.

Servings: 2

Prep Time: 10 minutes

Cook Time: 20 minutes

Total Time: 30 minutes

Nutrition Per Serving:

- **Calories:** 180
- **Protein:** 5g
- **Carbohydrates:** 15g
- **Fiber:** 4g
- **Fat:** 10g
- **Sodium:** 110mg

Ingredients:

✓ 1 cup broccoli florets
✓ ¼ cup raw almonds, chopped
✓ ½ small onion, diced
✓ 2 cups low-sodium vegetable broth
✓ 1 teaspoon olive oil
✓ ¼ teaspoon garlic powder
✓ ¼ teaspoon black pepper

Instructions:

1. Heat olive oil in a pot over medium heat.
2. Sauté onions for 3 minutes.
3. Add broccoli, almonds, garlic powder, and black pepper. Stir well.
4. Pour in vegetable broth and simmer for 15 minutes.
5. Blend the soup until smooth.

Cooking Tips:

✓ Toast the almonds before adding them for extra flavor.
✓ Garnish with a few almond slivers.

Health Benefits:

✓ **Broccoli** – Contains antioxidants that support joint health.
✓ **Almonds** – Provide healthy fats and vitamin E.

---

9. Cabbage and White Bean Soup

(Limit white beans to ½ cup per serving)

A high-fiber, heart-friendly soup that's easy on digestion.

Servings: 2

Prep Time: 10 minutes

Cook Time: 30 minutes

Total Time: 40 minutes

Nutrition Per Serving:

- **Calories:** 220
- **Protein:** 10g
- **Carbohydrates:** 38g
- **Fiber:** 10g
- **Fat:** 3g
- **Sodium:** 150mg

Ingredients:

✓ ½ cup cooked white beans

✓ 1 cup shredded cabbage

✓ ½ small onion, diced

✓ 1 carrot, diced

✓ 2 cups low-sodium vegetable broth

✓ 1 teaspoon olive oil

✓ ½ teaspoon thyme

✓ ¼ teaspoon black pepper

Instructions:

1. Heat olive oil in a pot over medium heat.
2. Sauté onions and carrots for 3 minutes.
3. Add cabbage, white beans, thyme, and black pepper. Stir well.
4. Pour in vegetable broth and simmer for 25 minutes.
5. Serve warm, garnished with fresh parsley.

Health Benefits:

✓ **Cabbage** – Supports gut health and reduces inflammation.

✓ **White Beans** – Provide plant-based protein and fiber.

---

10. Mushroom-Free Vegetable Barley Soup

A hearty, fiber-rich soup that's completely mushroom-free and gout-friendly.

Servings: 2

Prep Time: 10 minutes

Cook Time: 30 minutes

Total Time: 40 minutes

Nutrition Per Serving:

- **Calories:** 220
- **Protein:** 6g
- **Carbohydrates:** 40g
- **Fiber:** 8g
- **Fat:** 3g

- **Sodium:** 120mg

Ingredients:

✓ ½ cup pearl barley, rinsed

✓ 1 small carrot, diced

✓ ½ cup zucchini, chopped

✓ ½ small onion, diced

✓ 1 celery stalk, chopped

✓ 2 cups low-sodium vegetable broth

✓ 1 teaspoon olive oil

✓ ½ teaspoon dried thyme

✓ ¼ teaspoon black pepper

Instructions:

1. Heat olive oil in a pot over medium heat.
2. Sauté onions, carrots, and celery for 5 minutes.
3. Add barley, zucchini, thyme, and black pepper. Stir well.
4. Pour in vegetable broth and bring to a boil.
5. Reduce heat and simmer for 30 minutes until barley is tender.
6. Serve warm with fresh parsley garnish.

Cooking Tips:

✓ **For a heartier version, add cooked lentils (limited to ½ cup per serving).**

✓ **Adjust seasoning to taste with a squeeze of lemon juice.**

Health Benefits:

✓ **Barley** – A great low-purine grain rich in fiber.

✓ **Zucchini & Carrots** – Provide vitamins for joint support.

---

11. Zucchini and Leek Soup

A light, creamy, and refreshing soup with a mild onion-like flavor.

Servings: 2

Prep Time: 10 minutes

Cook Time: 25 minutes

Total Time: 35 minutes

Nutrition Per Serving:

- **Calories:** 190
- **Protein:** 4g
- **Carbohydrates:** 30g
- **Fiber:** 5g
- **Fat:** 4g

- **Sodium:** 110mg

Ingredients:

✓ 1 cup zucchini, chopped

✓ ½ small leek, chopped (white part only)

✓ ½ small onion, diced

✓ 2 cups low-sodium vegetable broth

✓ 1 teaspoon olive oil

✓ ½ teaspoon dried basil

✓ ¼ teaspoon black pepper

Instructions:

1. Heat olive oil in a pot over medium heat.
2. Sauté onions and leeks for 3 minutes.
3. Add zucchini, basil, and black pepper. Stir well.
4. Pour in vegetable broth and bring to a boil.
5. Reduce heat and simmer for 20 minutes.
6. Blend for a smooth texture and serve warm.

Cooking Tips:

✓ For extra creaminess, add a small amount of unsweetened almond milk.

✓ Garnish with fresh dill for extra flavor.

Health Benefits:

✓ **Leeks & Zucchini** – Support digestion and are anti-inflammatory.

✓ **Olive Oil** – Provides heart-healthy fats.

---

12. Green Pea and Mint Soup

A refreshing and mildly sweet soup perfect for a light meal.

Servings: 2

Prep Time: 10 minutes

Cook Time: 15 minutes

Total Time: 25 minutes

Nutrition Per Serving:

- **Calories:** 180
- **Protein:** 6g
- **Carbohydrates:** 28g
- **Fiber:** 6g
- **Fat:** 3g
- **Sodium:** 100mg

Ingredients:

✓ 1 cup green peas (fresh or frozen)

✓ ½ small onion, diced

✓ 2 cups low-sodium vegetable broth

✓ 1 teaspoon olive oil

- ✓ ½ teaspoon dried mint
- ✓ ¼ teaspoon black pepper

Instructions:

1. Heat olive oil in a pot over medium heat.
2. Sauté onions for 3 minutes.
3. Add peas, mint, and black pepper. Stir well.
4. Pour in vegetable broth and simmer for 10 minutes.
5. Blend for a smooth texture and serve warm.

Cooking Tips:

✓ Top with fresh mint leaves for a refreshing taste.

✓ Add a squeeze of lemon juice before serving.

Health Benefits:

✓ **Green Peas** – Contain plant-based protein and antioxidants.

✓ **Mint** – Supports digestion and reduces inflammation.

13. Spiced Apple and Carrot Soup

A slightly sweet and warming soup, rich in antioxidants.

Servings: 2

Prep Time: 10 minutes

Cook Time: 20 minutes

Total Time: 30 minutes

Ingredients:

- ✓ 1 apple, peeled and chopped
- ✓ 1 medium carrot, chopped
- ✓ ½ small onion, diced
- ✓ 2 cups low-sodium vegetable broth
- ✓ 1 teaspoon olive oil
- ✓ ½ teaspoon cinnamon
- ✓ ¼ teaspoon nutmeg

Instructions:

1. Sauté onions in olive oil for 3 minutes.
2. Add carrots, apple, cinnamon, and nutmeg. Stir well.
3. Pour in broth and simmer for 20 minutes.
4. Blend for a smooth texture and serve warm.

14. Tomato and Red Pepper Soup

A simple, flavorful soup packed with antioxidants.

Servings: 2

Prep Time: 10 minutes

Cook Time: 25 minutes

Total Time: 35 minutes

Ingredients:

- ✓ 1 cup diced tomatoes
- ✓ 1 red bell pepper, chopped
- ✓ ½ small onion, diced
- ✓ 2 cups low-sodium vegetable broth
- ✓ 1 teaspoon olive oil
- ✓ ½ teaspoon dried oregano
- ✓ ¼ teaspoon black pepper

Instructions:

1. Sauté onions and red bell pepper for 3 minutes.
2. Add tomatoes, oregano, and black pepper.
3. Pour in broth and simmer for 20 minutes.
4. Blend and serve warm.

15. Lemon Lentil Soup *(Limit lentils to ½ cup per serving)*

A comforting and protein-packed soup with a hint of citrus for freshness.

Servings: 2

Prep Time: 10 minutes

Cook Time: 30 minutes

Total Time: 40 minutes

Nutrition Per Serving:

- **Calories:** 220
- **Protein:** 12g
- **Carbohydrates:** 35g
- **Fiber:** 9g
- **Fat:** 3g
- **Sodium:** 120mg

Ingredients:

- ✓ ½ cup cooked lentils (moderation recommended for gout)
- ✓ ½ small onion, diced
- ✓ 1 small carrot, diced
- ✓ 2 cups low-sodium vegetable broth
- ✓ 1 teaspoon olive oil
- ✓ ½ teaspoon ground cumin

- ✓ ¼ teaspoon black pepper
- ✓ Juice of ½ lemon

Instructions:

1. Heat olive oil in a pot over medium heat.
2. Sauté onions and carrots for 3 minutes.
3. Add cooked lentils, cumin, and black pepper. Stir well.
4. Pour in vegetable broth and simmer for 25 minutes.
5. Stir in fresh lemon juice before serving.

Cooking Tips:

✓ Use red lentils for a smoother texture.
✓ Garnish with chopped parsley for extra freshness.

Health Benefits:

✓ **Lentils** – A good plant-based protein source but should be eaten in moderation.
✓ **Lemon Juice** – Helps alkalize the body and supports digestion.

16. Hearty Quinoa and Vegetable Stew

A filling, nutrient-dense stew that's gentle on the joints.

Servings: 2

Prep Time: 10 minutes

Cook Time: 30 minutes

Total Time: 40 minutes

Nutrition Per Serving:

- **Calories:** 250
- **Protein:** 8g
- **Carbohydrates:** 40g
- **Fiber:** 6g
- **Fat:** 5g
- **Sodium:** 115mg

Ingredients:

✓ ½ cup cooked quinoa
✓ ½ small onion, diced
✓ ½ cup zucchini, chopped
✓ ½ cup carrots, chopped
✓ ½ cup green beans, chopped
✓ 2 cups low-sodium vegetable broth
✓ 1 teaspoon olive oil

✓ ½ teaspoon dried thyme

✓ ¼ teaspoon black pepper

<u>Instructions:</u>

1. Heat olive oil in a pot over medium heat.
2. Sauté onions, zucchini, and carrots for 3 minutes.
3. Add green beans, cooked quinoa, thyme, and black pepper. Stir well.
4. Pour in vegetable broth and simmer for 25 minutes.
5. Serve warm with a sprinkle of fresh parsley.

<u>Cooking Tips:</u>

✓ For extra heartiness, add diced sweet potatoes.

✓ Quinoa is naturally gluten-free and easy to digest.

<u>Health Benefits:</u>

✓ **Quinoa** – A complete protein that is low in purines.

✓ **Zucchini & Carrots** – Provide vitamins and antioxidants.

17. Kale and Sweet Potato Stew

A fiber-rich and anti-inflammatory stew with a natural sweetness.

Servings: 2

Prep Time: 10 minutes

Cook Time: 25 minutes

Total Time: 35 minutes

<u>Nutrition Per Serving:</u>

- **Calories:** 230
- **Protein:** 7g
- **Carbohydrates:** 38g
- **Fiber:** 7g
- **Fat:** 4g
- **Sodium:** 100mg

<u>Ingredients:</u>

✓ ½ cup chopped sweet potato

✓ ½ cup chopped kale (moderation recommended)

✓ ½ small onion, diced

✓ ½ cup carrots, chopped

✓ 2 cups low-sodium vegetable broth

✓ 1 teaspoon olive oil

✓ ½ teaspoon ground turmeric

✓ ¼ teaspoon black pepper

Instructions:

1. Heat olive oil in a pot over medium heat.
2. Sauté onions and carrots for 3 minutes.
3. Add sweet potatoes, kale, turmeric, and black pepper. Stir well.
4. Pour in vegetable broth and simmer for 20 minutes.
5. Serve warm with a sprinkle of sesame seeds.

Cooking Tips:

✓ **For a creamier texture, blend half of the stew before serving.**
✓ **Kale should be consumed in moderation due to its purine content.**

Health Benefits:

✓ **Sweet Potatoes** – Provide fiber and anti-inflammatory nutrients.
✓ **Turmeric** – Has powerful anti-inflammatory properties.

18. Turmeric-Spiced Pumpkin Soup

A warm and healing soup packed with antioxidants.

Servings: 2

Prep Time: 10 minutes

Cook Time: 20 minutes

Total Time: 30 minutes

Nutrition Per Serving:

- **Calories:** 200
- **Protein:** 5g
- **Carbohydrates:** 32g
- **Fiber:** 6g
- **Fat:** 4g
- **Sodium:** 95mg

Ingredients:

✓ 1 cup pumpkin, chopped
✓ ½ small onion, diced
✓ ½ small carrot, diced
✓ 2 cups low-sodium vegetable broth
✓ 1 teaspoon olive oil
✓ ½ teaspoon ground turmeric
✓ ¼ teaspoon black pepper

Instructions:

1. Heat olive oil in a pot over medium heat.
2. Sauté onions and carrots for 3 minutes.
3. Add pumpkin, turmeric, and black pepper. Stir well.
4. Pour in vegetable broth and simmer for 20 minutes.
5. Blend until smooth and serve warm.

Cooking Tips:

✓ For extra creaminess, add a splash of unsweetened almond milk.

✓ Pair with whole-grain toast for a balanced meal.

Health Benefits:

✓ **Pumpkin** – A nutrient-dense, low-purine food.

✓ **Turmeric** – Reduces joint inflammation and supports digestion.

CHAPTER 6: GOUT-FRIENDLY SALADS & SIDES

1. Cucumber and Avocado Salad with Lemon Dressing

A light and refreshing salad that's hydrating and packed with healthy fats for joint health.

Servings: 2
Prep Time: 10 minutes
Total Time: 10 minutes

Nutrition Per Serving

- **Calories:** 180
- **Protein:** 2g
- **Carbohydrates:** 12g
- **Fiber:** 6g
- **Fat:** 14g
- **Sodium:** 30mg

Ingredients

- 1 large cucumber, sliced
- ½ ripe avocado, diced
- 1 tablespoon extra virgin olive oil
- 1 tablespoon fresh lemon juice
- ½ teaspoon honey (optional)
- 1 tablespoon fresh parsley, chopped
- ¼ teaspoon sea salt
- ¼ teaspoon black pepper

Instructions

1. Wash and slice the cucumber into thin rounds.
2. Dice the avocado into small cubes.
3. In a small bowl, whisk together the olive oil, lemon juice, honey (if using), salt, and pepper.
4. Combine cucumber and avocado in a salad bowl.
5. Drizzle with the dressing and gently toss to coat.
6. Sprinkle fresh parsley on top and serve immediately.

Cooking Tips

- Serve chilled for extra freshness.
- Add a sprinkle of flaxseeds for additional omega-3 benefits.

Health Benefits

- **Cucumber** is hydrating and helps flush out excess uric acid.

- **Avocado** provides heart-healthy monounsaturated fats, supporting joint lubrication.

---

2. Zucchini Noodles with Pesto

A light and nutritious alternative to pasta with a delicious basil-almond pesto.

Servings: 2
Prep Time: 15 minutes
Total Time: 15 minutes

Nutrition Per Serving

- **Calories:** 220
- **Protein:** 5g
- **Carbohydrates:** 10g
- **Fiber:** 4g
- **Fat:** 18g
- **Sodium:** 40mg

Ingredients

- 2 medium zucchinis, spiralized
- ¼ cup fresh basil leaves
- 2 tablespoons almonds (unsalted)
- 1 tablespoon extra virgin olive oil
- 1 tablespoon lemon juice
- 1 garlic clove, minced
- ¼ teaspoon sea salt
- ¼ teaspoon black pepper

Instructions

1. Spiralize the zucchinis into noodle-like strands.
2. In a food processor, blend basil, almonds, olive oil, lemon juice, garlic, salt, and pepper until smooth.
3. Toss the zucchini noodles with the pesto sauce.
4. Serve immediately or chill before serving.

Cooking Tips

- If you prefer warm noodles, lightly sauté the zucchini for 1–2 minutes.
- Add a sprinkle of nutritional yeast for a cheesy flavor.

Health Benefits

- **Zucchini** is hydrating and helps lower inflammation.
- **Almonds** provide anti-inflammatory fats and vitamin E for joint health.

3. Carrot and Apple Slaw

A crunchy, refreshing slaw packed with antioxidants and gut-friendly fiber.

Servings: 2
Prep Time: 10 minutes
Total Time: 10 minutes

Nutrition Per Serving

- **Calories:** 150
- **Protein:** 2g
- **Carbohydrates:** 22g
- **Fiber:** 5g
- **Fat:** 7g
- **Sodium:** 40mg

Ingredients

- 1 large carrot, grated
- ½ medium apple, julienned
- 1 tablespoon fresh lemon juice
- 1 tablespoon extra virgin olive oil
- 1 teaspoon honey (optional)
- 1 tablespoon unsalted sunflower seeds
- ¼ teaspoon sea salt
- ¼ teaspoon black pepper

Instructions

1. In a mixing bowl, combine grated carrot and julienned apple.
2. In a small bowl, whisk together lemon juice, olive oil, honey (if using), salt, and pepper.
3. Drizzle the dressing over the carrot and apple mixture.
4. Toss well to coat evenly.
5. Sprinkle with sunflower seeds before serving.

Cooking Tips

- Use a mandoline slicer for quick and even julienne cuts.
- If preparing in advance, add lemon juice last to prevent apple from browning.

Health Benefits

- **Carrots** provide beta-carotene, which reduces inflammation.
- **Apples** contain polyphenols that help lower uric acid levels.

4. Quinoa and Kale Salad with Citrus Dressing

A protein-rich, anti-inflammatory salad to support joint health.

Servings: 2
Prep Time: 15 minutes
Cook Time: 10 minutes
Total Time: 25 minutes

Nutrition Per Serving

- **Calories:** 210
- **Protein:** 7g
- **Carbohydrates:** 28g
- **Fiber:** 5g
- **Fat:** 8g
- **Sodium:** 35mg

Ingredients

- ½ cup cooked quinoa
- 1 cup chopped kale (massaged with lemon juice)
- ½ orange, segmented
- 1 tablespoon pumpkin seeds
- 1 tablespoon extra virgin olive oil
- 1 tablespoon fresh lemon juice
- ½ teaspoon Dijon mustard
- ¼ teaspoon sea salt
- ¼ teaspoon black pepper

Instructions

1. Cook quinoa according to package instructions and let cool.
2. In a large bowl, massage the chopped kale with lemon juice to soften it.
3. Add cooked quinoa, orange segments, and pumpkin seeds.
4. In a separate bowl, whisk together olive oil, lemon juice, Dijon mustard, salt, and pepper.
5. Drizzle dressing over the salad and toss to combine.
6. Serve chilled or at room temperature.

Cooking Tips

- Massage kale for 2–3 minutes to reduce bitterness.
- Use red quinoa for extra antioxidants.

Health Benefits

- **Quinoa** is a complete protein with anti-inflammatory properties.
- **Kale** provides vitamin C, which supports collagen production for healthy joints.

5. Steamed Green Beans with Almonds

A simple, nutrient-dense side dish that fights inflammation.

Servings: 2
Prep Time: 5 minutes
Cook Time: 8 minutes
Total Time: 13 minutes

Nutrition Per Serving

- **Calories:** 130
- **Protein:** 4g
- **Carbohydrates:** 12g
- **Fiber:** 5g
- **Fat:** 7g
- **Sodium:** 25mg

Ingredients

- 1 cup fresh green beans, trimmed
- 1 tablespoon sliced almonds
- 1 teaspoon extra virgin olive oil
- ½ teaspoon lemon zest
- ¼ teaspoon sea salt
- ¼ teaspoon black pepper

Instructions

1. Steam green beans for 5–7 minutes until tender-crisp.
2. In a dry skillet, toast almonds over low heat for 2 minutes.
3. Toss the steamed green beans with olive oil, salt, and pepper.
4. Top with toasted almonds and lemon zest before serving.

Cooking Tips

- Avoid overcooking the green beans to preserve nutrients.
- Use slivered almonds for extra crunch.

Health Benefits

- **Green beans** provide vitamin K and fiber for joint support.
- **Almonds** offer vitamin E, which reduces inflammation.

---

6. Roasted Sweet Potatoes with Garlic

A naturally sweet, anti-inflammatory side dish to support joint health.

Servings: 2
Prep Time: 10 minutes

Cook Time: 25 minutes
Total Time: 35 minutes

Nutrition Per Serving

- **Calories:** 180
- **Protein:** 2g
- **Carbohydrates:** 35g
- **Fiber:** 5g
- **Fat:** 5g
- **Sodium:** 40mg

Ingredients

- 1 medium sweet potato, peeled and cubed
- 1 tablespoon extra virgin olive oil
- 1 teaspoon minced garlic
- ½ teaspoon paprika
- ¼ teaspoon sea salt
- ¼ teaspoon black pepper

Instructions

1. Preheat the oven to 400°F (200°C).
2. In a mixing bowl, toss sweet potato cubes with olive oil, garlic, paprika, salt, and pepper.
3. Spread the sweet potatoes evenly on a baking sheet.
4. Roast for 25 minutes, stirring halfway through, until tender and slightly crispy.
5. Serve warm as a delicious side.

Cooking Tips

- Use parchment paper for easy cleanup.
- Roast at a high temperature for caramelization and natural sweetness.

Health Benefits

- **Sweet potatoes** are rich in antioxidants and fiber, reducing inflammation.
- **Garlic** has natural anti-inflammatory properties, helping with joint pain.

---

7. Pumpkin and Spinach Salad with Goat Cheese

A flavorful, nutrient-packed salad with a touch of creaminess.

Servings: 2
Prep Time: 10 minutes
Cook Time: 20 minutes
Total Time: 30 minutes

Nutrition Per Serving

- **Calories:** 220
- **Protein:** 7g
- **Carbohydrates:** 28g
- **Fiber:** 6g
- **Fat:** 9g
- **Sodium:** 100mg

Ingredients

- 1 cup diced pumpkin
- 1 teaspoon extra virgin olive oil
- 1 cup fresh spinach (Spinach in moderation)
- 2 tablespoons crumbled goat cheese
- 1 tablespoon pumpkin seeds
- ½ tablespoon balsamic vinegar
- ¼ teaspoon sea salt
- ¼ teaspoon black pepper

Instructions

1. Preheat the oven to 375°F (190°C).
2. Toss diced pumpkin with olive oil, salt, and pepper. Roast for 20 minutes until tender.
3. In a bowl, combine spinach, roasted pumpkin, and crumbled goat cheese.
4. Drizzle with balsamic vinegar and sprinkle with pumpkin seeds.
5. Serve immediately.

Cooking Tips

- Allow roasted pumpkin to cool slightly before adding to the salad.
- Replace goat cheese with feta for a saltier option.

Health Benefits

- **Pumpkin** provides beta-carotene, which helps reduce inflammation.
- **Goat cheese** is a lower-fat, lower-purine cheese alternative.

---

8. Broccoli and Carrot Slaw

A crunchy and fiber-rich slaw that supports digestion and joint health.

Servings: 2
Prep Time: 10 minutes
Total Time: 10 minutes

Nutrition Per Serving

- **Calories:** 140
- **Protein:** 4g
- **Carbohydrates:** 18g
- **Fiber:** 6g

- **Fat:** 6g
- **Sodium:** 35mg

Ingredients

- 1 cup shredded broccoli
- ½ cup grated carrot
- 1 tablespoon extra virgin olive oil
- 1 tablespoon apple cider vinegar
- ½ teaspoon Dijon mustard
- ¼ teaspoon sea salt
- ¼ teaspoon black pepper

Instructions

1. In a mixing bowl, combine shredded broccoli and grated carrot.
2. In a small bowl, whisk together olive oil, apple cider vinegar, Dijon mustard, salt, and pepper.
3. Drizzle dressing over the slaw and toss well.
4. Let sit for 5 minutes before serving to absorb flavors.

Cooking Tips

- Use a food processor to quickly shred broccoli.
- Allow the slaw to marinate longer for better flavor.

Health Benefits

- **Broccoli** is rich in fiber and vitamin C, reducing oxidative stress.
- **Carrots** add anti-inflammatory properties and improve digestion.

---

9. Tomato and Bell Pepper Salad with Olive Oil

A refreshing, vitamin-packed salad perfect for a light meal.

Servings: 2
Prep Time: 10 minutes
Total Time: 10 minutes

Nutrition Per Serving

- **Calories:** 120
- **Protein:** 2g
- **Carbohydrates:** 14g
- **Fiber:** 4g
- **Fat:** 6g
- **Sodium:** 25mg

Ingredients

- 1 cup cherry tomatoes, halved
- ½ red bell pepper, diced
- ½ yellow bell pepper, diced

- 1 tablespoon extra virgin olive oil
- 1 teaspoon fresh lemon juice
- ¼ teaspoon sea salt
- ¼ teaspoon black pepper

Instructions

1. In a bowl, combine cherry tomatoes and diced bell peppers.
2. Drizzle with olive oil and lemon juice.
3. Season with salt and pepper, then toss gently.
4. Serve immediately.

Cooking Tips

- Use multicolored bell peppers for visual appeal and variety.
- Refrigerate for 15 minutes before serving for extra freshness.

Health Benefits

- **Tomatoes** provide lycopene, which reduces inflammation.
- **Bell peppers** are high in vitamin C, promoting joint health.

10. Steamed Brussels Sprouts with Lemon

A light and nutritious side dish rich in vitamins and antioxidants.

Servings: 2
Prep Time: 5 minutes
Cook Time: 10 minutes
Total Time: 15 minutes

Nutrition Per Serving

- **Calories:** 80
- **Protein:** 4g
- **Carbohydrates:** 14g
- **Fiber:** 5g
- **Fat:** 2g
- **Sodium:** 15mg

Ingredients

- 1 cup Brussels sprouts, trimmed and halved
- 1 teaspoon extra virgin olive oil
- 1 teaspoon fresh lemon juice
- ¼ teaspoon sea salt
- ¼ teaspoon black pepper

Instructions

1. Bring a pot of water to a boil and place a steamer basket inside.

2. Add Brussels sprouts to the steamer basket and cover.
3. Steam for 8–10 minutes until tender but still firm.
4. Transfer to a bowl and toss with olive oil, lemon juice, salt, and pepper.
5. Serve warm as a side dish.

Cooking Tips

- Avoid overcooking to prevent bitterness.
- Roast for a crispier texture instead of steaming.

Health Benefits

- **Brussels sprouts** are high in antioxidants and fiber, helping reduce inflammation.
- **Lemon juice** enhances digestion and alkalizes the body.

---

11. Cauliflower Mash with Garlic

(Limited to ½ cup per serving)

A creamy, low-carb alternative to mashed potatoes, perfect for joint health.

Servings: 2
Prep Time: 10 minutes
Cook Time: 10 minutes
Total Time: 20 minutes

Nutrition Per Serving

- **Calories:** 90
- **Protein:** 3g
- **Carbohydrates:** 12g
- **Fiber:** 4g
- **Fat:** 4g
- **Sodium:** 20mg

Ingredients

- 1 cup cauliflower florets (use only ½ cup per serving)
- 1 teaspoon extra virgin olive oil
- ½ teaspoon minced garlic
- 2 tablespoons unsweetened almond milk
- ¼ teaspoon sea salt
- ¼ teaspoon black pepper

Instructions

1. Steam the cauliflower florets for 8–10 minutes until soft.
2. Transfer to a food processor and add olive oil, garlic, almond milk, salt, and pepper.

3. Blend until smooth and creamy.
4. Serve warm as a side dish.

Cooking Tips

- Adjust almond milk for desired consistency.
- Add a pinch of turmeric for extra anti-inflammatory benefits.

Health Benefits

- **Cauliflower** provides fiber and antioxidants but should be eaten in moderation.
- **Garlic** has natural anti-inflammatory and immune-boosting properties.

---

12. Warm Beet and Walnut Salad

A vibrant and heart-healthy salad packed with antioxidants.

Servings: 2
Prep Time: 10 minutes
Cook Time: 25 minutes
Total Time: 35 minutes

Nutrition Per Serving

- **Calories:** 170
- **Protein:** 5g
- **Carbohydrates:** 20g
- **Fiber:** 6g
- **Fat:** 8g
- **Sodium:** 50mg

Ingredients

- 1 medium beet, peeled and diced
- 1 teaspoon extra virgin olive oil
- 1 tablespoon walnuts, chopped
- ½ teaspoon balsamic vinegar
- ¼ teaspoon sea salt
- ¼ teaspoon black pepper

Instructions

1. Preheat the oven to 375°F (190°C).
2. Toss diced beet with olive oil, salt, and pepper.
3. Roast for 25 minutes until tender.
4. Let cool slightly, then mix with walnuts and balsamic vinegar.
5. Serve warm as a salad or side dish.

Cooking Tips

- Roast beets in foil to retain moisture.
- Use apple cider vinegar for a tangier flavor.

Health Benefits

- **Beets** help improve circulation and reduce inflammation.
- **Walnuts** contain omega-3s that support joint health.

---

13. Grilled Zucchini and Red Pepper Salad

A simple, flavorful dish loaded with vitamins.

Servings: 2
Prep Time: 10 minutes
Cook Time: 10 minutes
Total Time: 20 minutes

Nutrition Per Serving

- **Calories:** 90
- **Protein:** 3g
- **Carbohydrates:** 15g
- **Fiber:** 5g
- **Fat:** 3g
- **Sodium:** 30mg

Ingredients

- 1 small zucchini, sliced
- ½ red bell pepper, sliced
- 1 teaspoon extra virgin olive oil
- ½ teaspoon fresh lemon juice
- ¼ teaspoon sea salt
- ¼ teaspoon black pepper

Instructions

1. Preheat a grill pan over medium heat.
2. Brush zucchini and red pepper slices with olive oil and season with salt and pepper.
3. Grill for 3–4 minutes per side until tender and lightly charred.
4. Remove from heat and drizzle with lemon juice.
5. Serve as a warm salad or side dish.

Cooking Tips

- Use an outdoor grill for a smoky flavor.
- Add fresh herbs like basil or parsley for extra taste.

Health Benefits

- **Zucchini** is hydrating and low in purines.
- **Red peppers** are rich in vitamin C, helping protect joints.

14. Quinoa and Roasted Vegetable Medley

A protein-rich and fiber-packed side dish that's easy on the joints.

Servings: 2
Prep Time: 10 minutes
Cook Time: 20 minutes
Total Time: 30 minutes

Nutrition Per Serving

- **Calories:** 180
- **Protein:** 6g
- **Carbohydrates:** 28g
- **Fiber:** 5g
- **Fat:** 5g
- **Sodium:** 40mg

Ingredients

- ½ cup cooked quinoa
- ½ zucchini, diced
- ½ red bell pepper, diced
- ½ cup cherry tomatoes, halved
- 1 teaspoon extra virgin olive oil
- ½ teaspoon dried oregano
- ¼ teaspoon sea salt
- ¼ teaspoon black pepper

Instructions

1. Preheat the oven to 400°F (200°C).
2. Toss zucchini, bell pepper, and cherry tomatoes with olive oil, oregano, salt, and pepper.
3. Spread the vegetables on a baking sheet and roast for 15–20 minutes, until tender.
4. In a bowl, combine cooked quinoa with roasted vegetables.
5. Serve warm as a side dish.

Cooking Tips

- Use tricolor quinoa for extra texture.
- Squeeze fresh lemon juice on top for added flavor.

Health Benefits

- **Quinoa** is a complete protein that is low in purines.
- **Roasted vegetables** provide antioxidants that reduce inflammation.

15. Carrot and Parsnip Mash

A naturally sweet and creamy alternative to mashed potatoes.

Servings: 2
Prep Time: 10 minutes
Cook Time: 15 minutes
Total Time: 25 minutes

Nutrition Per Serving

- **Calories:** 130
- **Protein:** 2g
- **Carbohydrates:** 30g
- **Fiber:** 6g
- **Fat:** 2g
- **Sodium:** 25mg

Ingredients

- 1 medium carrot, peeled and chopped
- 1 medium parsnip, peeled and chopped
- ½ teaspoon extra virgin olive oil
- 1 tablespoon unsweetened almond milk
- ¼ teaspoon sea salt
- ¼ teaspoon black pepper

Instructions

1. Boil carrot and parsnip pieces in water for 12–15 minutes, until tender.
2. Drain and transfer to a bowl.
3. Mash with a fork or blend with olive oil, almond milk, salt, and pepper until smooth.
4. Serve warm as a side dish.

Cooking Tips

- For a richer texture, use a food processor instead of mashing by hand.
- Add a pinch of nutmeg for a warm flavor.

Health Benefits

- **Carrots** and **parsnips** are high in fiber and support digestion.
- **Olive oil** adds healthy fats that fight inflammation.

16. Lettuce Wraps with Avocado and Chickpea Filling (Limit chickpeas to ½ cup per serving)

A fresh and nutritious wrap that's perfect as a side or light meal.

Servings: 2
Prep Time: 10 minutes
Total Time: 10 minutes

Nutrition Per Serving

- **Calories:** 200
- **Protein:** 7g
- **Carbohydrates:** 25g
- **Fiber:** 8g
- **Fat:** 9g
- **Sodium:** 35mg

Ingredients

- 4 large lettuce leaves
- ½ cup cooked chickpeas (use only ¼ cup per serving)
- ½ avocado, mashed
- ½ teaspoon lemon juice
- ¼ teaspoon garlic powder
- ¼ teaspoon sea salt
- ¼ teaspoon black pepper

Instructions

1. In a bowl, mash chickpeas with avocado, lemon juice, garlic powder, salt, and pepper.
2. Spoon the mixture onto lettuce leaves.
3. Fold the leaves and serve as wraps.

Cooking Tips

- Use butter lettuce for the best wrap texture.
- Add diced cucumber for extra crunch.

Health Benefits

- **Chickpeas** provide plant-based protein but should be eaten in moderation.
- **Avocado** adds heart-healthy fats that help reduce inflammation.

---

17. Roasted Cabbage with Olive Oil

A crispy, flavorful side dish packed with fiber and vitamins.

Servings: 2
Prep Time: 5 minutes

Cook Time: 20 minutes

Total Time: 25 minutes

Nutrition Per Serving

- **Calories:** 90
- **Protein:** 2g
- **Carbohydrates:** 12g
- **Fiber:** 5g
- **Fat:** 4g
- **Sodium:** 30mg

Ingredients

- 2 cups cabbage, sliced into wedges
- 1 teaspoon extra virgin olive oil
- ¼ teaspoon sea salt
- ¼ teaspoon black pepper

Instructions

1. Preheat the oven to 400°F (200°C).
2. Place cabbage wedges on a baking sheet and brush with olive oil.
3. Sprinkle with salt and pepper.
4. Roast for 20 minutes, turning halfway, until crispy and slightly caramelized.
5. Serve warm as a side dish.

Cooking Tips

- Roast at a higher temperature for extra crispiness.
- Add a squeeze of lemon juice for a fresh twist.

Health Benefits

- **Cabbage** is rich in antioxidants and supports digestion.
- **Olive oil** provides anti-inflammatory benefits.

---

18. Butternut Squash and Kale Side Dish

A nutrient-dense, anti-inflammatory dish rich in vitamins.

Servings: 2
Prep Time: 10 minutes
Cook Time: 20 minutes
Total Time: 30 minutes

Nutrition Per Serving

- **Calories:** 140
- **Protein:** 4g
- **Carbohydrates:** 28g
- **Fiber:** 6g
- **Fat:** 3g

- **Sodium:** 40mg

Ingredients

- 1 cup butternut squash, diced
- 1 cup kale, chopped
- 1 teaspoon extra virgin olive oil
- ½ teaspoon garlic powder
- ¼ teaspoon sea salt
- ¼ teaspoon black pepper

Instructions

1. Preheat the oven to 400°F (200°C).
2. Toss butternut squash with olive oil, garlic powder, salt, and pepper.
3. Roast for 15 minutes until tender.
4. In a pan, sauté kale over medium heat for 3 minutes until slightly wilted.
5. Mix kale with roasted butternut squash and serve warm.

Cooking Tips

- Massage kale with olive oil before cooking to make it tender.
- Sprinkle with pumpkin seeds for extra crunch.

Health Benefits

- **Butternut squash** is rich in vitamin A and helps reduce inflammation.
- **Kale** provides antioxidants but should be eaten in moderation.

CHAPTER 7: LOW-PURINE SNACKS & SMALL BITES

1. Baked Sweet Potato Fries

A crispy and nutritious snack rich in fiber and antioxidants.

Servings: 2
Prep Time: 10 minutes
Cook Time: 20 minutes
Total Time: 30 minutes

Nutrition Per Serving

- **Calories:** 180
- **Protein:** 3g
- **Carbohydrates:** 36g
- **Fiber:** 5g
- **Fat:** 4g
- **Sodium:** 80mg

Ingredients

- 1 medium sweet potato, cut into thin fries
- 1 teaspoon extra virgin olive oil
- ½ teaspoon paprika
- ¼ teaspoon garlic powder
- ¼ teaspoon sea salt

Instructions

1. Preheat oven to 425°F (220°C).
2. Toss sweet potato fries with olive oil, paprika, garlic powder, and salt.
3. Spread fries in a single layer on a baking sheet lined with parchment paper.
4. Bake for 20 minutes, flipping halfway through, until crispy and golden.
5. Serve warm.

Cooking Tips

- For extra crispiness, soak the sweet potato slices in water for 30 minutes before baking.
- Sprinkle with a dash of cinnamon for a sweet variation.

Health Benefits

- **Sweet potatoes** are low in purines and packed with anti-inflammatory compounds.

2. Carrot and Hummus Sticks

(Limit hummus portions)

A crunchy and protein-rich snack.

Servings: 2
Prep Time: 5 minutes
Total Time: 5 minutes

Nutrition Per Serving

- **Calories:** 160
- **Protein:** 4g
- **Carbohydrates:** 18g
- **Fiber:** 5g
- **Fat:** 8g
- **Sodium:** 100mg

Ingredients

- 1 medium carrot, cut into sticks
- ¼ cup hummus (limit to 2 tablespoons per serving)

Instructions

1. Slice the carrot into thin sticks.
2. Serve with a small portion of hummus for dipping.

Cooking Tips

- Use homemade hummus with tahini for a healthier version.
- Replace carrots with cucumber or celery for variety.

Health Benefits

- **Carrots** are high in fiber and antioxidants that support digestion.
- **Hummus (in moderation)** provides plant-based protein and healthy fats.

---

3. Cucumber and Avocado Roll-Ups

A refreshing, creamy, and low-purine snack.

Servings: 2
Prep Time: 10 minutes
Total Time: 10 minutes

Nutrition Per Serving

- **Calories:** 140
- **Protein:** 2g
- **Carbohydrates:** 10g
- **Fiber:** 5g
- **Fat:** 10g
- **Sodium:** 20mg

Ingredients

- 1 medium cucumber, thinly sliced lengthwise
- ½ avocado, mashed

- ½ teaspoon lemon juice
- ¼ teaspoon garlic powder
- ¼ teaspoon sea salt

Instructions

1. Lay out cucumber slices on a flat surface.
2. In a bowl, mix mashed avocado with lemon juice, garlic powder, and salt.
3. Spread a thin layer of avocado mixture onto each cucumber slice.
4. Roll up each slice and secure with a toothpick if needed.
5. Serve immediately.

Cooking Tips

- Chill the roll-ups for 10 minutes before serving for a firmer texture.
- Sprinkle with black sesame seeds for extra crunch.

Health Benefits

- **Cucumbers** are hydrating and support kidney health.
- **Avocado** provides heart-healthy fats and reduces inflammation.

4. Quinoa Crackers with Guacamole

A crunchy, gluten-free snack with healthy fats.

Servings: 2
Prep Time: 15 minutes
Cook Time: 15 minutes
Total Time: 30 minutes

Nutrition Per Serving

- **Calories:** 190
- **Protein:** 5g
- **Carbohydrates:** 24g
- **Fiber:** 6g
- **Fat:** 9g
- **Sodium:** 30mg

Ingredients

For the Crackers:

- ½ cup cooked quinoa
- 2 tablespoons ground flaxseed
- ½ teaspoon dried oregano
- ¼ teaspoon sea salt

For the Guacamole:

- ½ avocado, mashed
- ½ teaspoon lime juice

- ¼ teaspoon garlic powder

Instructions

1. Preheat oven to 350°F (175°C).
2. Mix quinoa, flaxseed, oregano, and salt in a bowl.
3. Press the mixture into a thin layer on a lined baking sheet.
4. Bake for 12–15 minutes until crisp, then break into pieces.
5. Serve with guacamole.

Cooking Tips

- Store crackers in an airtight container for up to a week.
- Add chili flakes for a spicy kick.

Health Benefits

- **Quinoa** is a complete protein and low in purines.
- **Avocado** supports joint and heart health.

5. Almond Butter and Apple Slices

A naturally sweet and satisfying snack.

Servings: 2
Prep Time: 5 minutes
Total Time: 5 minutes

Nutrition Per Serving

- **Calories:** 170
- **Protein:** 4g
- **Carbohydrates:** 22g
- **Fiber:** 5g
- **Fat:** 8g
- **Sodium:** 0mg

Ingredients

- 1 medium apple, sliced
- 2 tablespoons almond butter

Instructions

1. Slice the apple into thin wedges.
2. Spread almond butter on each slice.
3. Serve immediately.

Cooking Tips

- Sprinkle cinnamon on top for extra flavor.

- Use a crisp apple variety like Honeycrisp or Fuji.

Health Benefits

- **Apples** provide fiber and natural sweetness.
- **Almond butter** is rich in healthy fats and vitamin E.

---

6. Steamed Edamame with Sea Salt (Limit to ½ cup per serving)

A protein-packed, low-purine snack.

Servings: 2
Prep Time: 5 minutes
Cook Time: 5 minutes
Total Time: 10 minutes

Nutrition Per Serving

- **Calories:** 120
- **Protein:** 10g
- **Carbohydrates:** 9g
- **Fiber:** 4g
- **Fat:** 5g
- **Sodium:** 50mg

Ingredients

- ½ cup steamed edamame
- ¼ teaspoon sea salt

Instructions

1. Bring a pot of water to a boil.
2. Add edamame and boil for 5 minutes.
3. Drain, sprinkle with sea salt, and serve warm.

Cooking Tips

- Add a squeeze of lemon for a citrusy touch.
- Enjoy cold for a refreshing snack.

Health Benefits

- **Edamame** provides plant-based protein and fiber.
- **Sea salt** enhances flavor without increasing uric acid.

---

7. Zucchini Chips with Paprika

A crispy, low-calorie snack packed with antioxidants.

Servings: 2
Prep Time: 10 minutes
Cook Time: 30 minutes
Total Time: 40 minutes

Nutrition Per Serving

- **Calories:** 80
- **Protein:** 2g
- **Carbohydrates:** 12g
- **Fiber:** 3g
- **Fat:** 3g
- **Sodium:** 40mg

Ingredients

- 1 medium zucchini, thinly sliced
- 1 teaspoon extra virgin olive oil
- ½ teaspoon paprika
- ¼ teaspoon sea salt

Instructions

1. Preheat oven to 250°F (120°C).
2. Toss zucchini slices with olive oil, paprika, and salt.
3. Spread slices in a single layer on a baking sheet lined with parchment paper.
4. Bake for 30–35 minutes, flipping halfway through, until crisp.
5. Serve immediately.

Cooking Tips

- Use a mandoline slicer for even, thin slices.
- Store in an airtight container to maintain crispness.

Health Benefits

- **Zucchini** is hydrating and supports digestive health.
- **Paprika** contains antioxidants that reduce inflammation.

---

8. Roasted Chickpeas with Turmeric (Limit to ½ cup per serving)

A crunchy and protein-rich snack with anti-inflammatory properties.

Servings: 2
Prep Time: 5 minutes
Cook Time: 30 minutes
Total Time: 35 minutes

Nutrition Per Serving

- **Calories:** 150
- **Protein:** 6g
- **Carbohydrates:** 24g
- **Fiber:** 6g
- **Fat:** 3g

- **Sodium:** 50mg

Ingredients

- ½ cup cooked chickpeas (drained and rinsed if canned)
- 1 teaspoon olive oil
- ½ teaspoon turmeric
- ¼ teaspoon garlic powder
- ¼ teaspoon sea salt

Instructions

1. Preheat oven to 375°F (190°C).
2. Toss chickpeas with olive oil, turmeric, garlic powder, and salt.
3. Spread on a baking sheet and bake for 25–30 minutes until crispy.
4. Let cool slightly and enjoy.

Cooking Tips

- Store in an airtight container for up to 3 days.
- Add a pinch of cayenne for a spicy twist.

Health Benefits

- **Chickpeas (in moderation)** offer plant-based protein.
- **Turmeric** contains curcumin, which reduces inflammation.

9. Pumpkin Seed Trail Mix (Limit portions)

A nutrient-dense, crunchy snack with healthy fats.

Servings: 2
Prep Time: 5 minutes
Total Time: 5 minutes

Nutrition Per Serving

- **Calories:** 180
- **Protein:** 6g
- **Carbohydrates:** 14g
- **Fiber:** 3g
- **Fat:** 12g
- **Sodium:** 20mg

Ingredients

- 2 tablespoons pumpkin seeds
- 2 tablespoons unsweetened coconut flakes
- 1 tablespoon almonds (chopped)
- 1 tablespoon dried cranberries (unsweetened)

Instructions

1. Combine all ingredients in a bowl.
2. Mix well and serve as a snack.

Cooking Tips

- Store in an airtight container for up to a week.
- Use sunflower seeds instead of almonds for variation.

Health Benefits

- **Pumpkin seeds** are high in magnesium, which supports bone health.
- **Cranberries** contain antioxidants that reduce inflammation.

---

10. Carrot and Ginger Energy Bites

A naturally sweet, no-bake snack packed with anti-inflammatory nutrients.

Servings: 6 bites
Prep Time: 10 minutes
Chill Time: 30 minutes
Total Time: 40 minutes

Nutrition Per Serving

- **Calories:** 120
- **Protein:** 3g
- **Carbohydrates:** 15g
- **Fiber:** 3g
- **Fat:** 6g
- **Sodium:** 10mg

Ingredients

- ½ cup rolled oats
- ¼ cup shredded carrot
- 1 tablespoon almond butter
- 1 tablespoon honey
- ½ teaspoon ground ginger
- 1 tablespoon chia seeds

Instructions

1. In a bowl, mix all ingredients until well combined.
2. Roll into small balls and place on a lined tray.
3. Refrigerate for at least 30 minutes before serving.

Cooking Tips

- Store in the fridge for up to a week.
- Substitute almond butter with sunflower seed butter for variation.

Health Benefits

- **Carrots** provide beta-carotene, which supports immune health.

11. Frozen Banana and Almond Butter Bites

A naturally sweet, refreshing snack with healthy fats.

Servings: 2
Prep Time: 5 minutes
Freeze Time: 1 hour
Total Time: 1 hour 5 minutes

Nutrition Per Serving

- **Calories:** 160
- **Protein:** 3g
- **Carbohydrates:** 25g
- **Fiber:** 4g
- **Fat:** 6g
- **Sodium:** 0mg

Ingredients

- 1 medium banana, sliced
- 2 tablespoons almond butter

Instructions

1. Spread almond butter on half of the banana slices.
2. Top with remaining banana slices to form mini sandwiches.
3. Place on a tray and freeze for at least 1 hour.
4. Serve frozen.

Cooking Tips

- Use peanut butter alternative if needed.
- Sprinkle with cinnamon for extra flavor.

Health Benefits

- **Bananas** support muscle function and reduce cramping.
- **Almond butter** provides vitamin E for joint health.

---

12. Coconut Yogurt with Chia Seeds

A creamy and gut-friendly snack rich in omega-3s.

Servings: 2
Prep Time: 5 minutes
Chill Time: 10 minutes
Total Time: 15 minutes

Nutrition Per Serving

- **Calories:** 140
- **Protein:** 3g
- **Carbohydrates:** 12g
- **Fiber:** 4g

- **Fat:** 8g
- **Sodium:** 20mg

Ingredients

- ½ cup unsweetened coconut yogurt
- 1 tablespoon chia seeds
- 1 teaspoon honey
- ½ teaspoon vanilla extract

Instructions

1. In a bowl, mix all ingredients together.
2. Let sit for 10 minutes to allow chia seeds to absorb liquid.
3. Serve chilled.

Cooking Tips

- Add sliced fruit like strawberries for extra flavor.
- Stir in a pinch of cinnamon for warmth.

Health Benefits

- **Chia seeds** are rich in omega-3s, which reduce inflammation.
- **Coconut yogurt** contains probiotics for gut health.

13. Homemade Quinoa Granola Bars

A crunchy, energy-packed snack that's perfect for on-the-go.

Servings: 6 bars
Prep Time: 10 minutes
Cook Time: 15 minutes
Total Time: 25 minutes

Nutrition Per Serving

- **Calories:** 180
- **Protein:** 5g
- **Carbohydrates:** 22g
- **Fiber:** 3g
- **Fat:** 8g
- **Sodium:** 30mg

Ingredients

- ½ cup cooked quinoa
- 1 cup rolled oats
- 2 tablespoons almond butter
- 2 tablespoons honey or maple syrup
- 1 teaspoon vanilla extract
- 2 tablespoons chopped walnuts (limit portions)

Instructions

1. Preheat oven to 350°F (175°C) and line a baking dish with parchment paper.
2. In a bowl, mix all ingredients until well combined.
3. Press the mixture into the prepared baking dish and bake for 15 minutes.
4. Let cool completely before cutting into bars.

Cooking Tips

- Store in an airtight container for up to a week.
- Add a sprinkle of cinnamon for extra warmth.

Health Benefits

- **Quinoa** is a complete protein that supports muscle health.
- **Walnuts (in moderation)** provide omega-3 fatty acids that reduce inflammation.

14. Baked Apple Chips with Cinnamon

A naturally sweet, crispy snack rich in antioxidants.

Servings: 2
Prep Time: 5 minutes
Cook Time: 2 hours
Total Time: 2 hours 5 minutes

Nutrition Per Serving

- **Calories:** 90
- **Protein:** 0.5g
- **Carbohydrates:** 24g
- **Fiber:** 4g
- **Fat:** 0g
- **Sodium:** 0mg

Ingredients

- 1 large apple, thinly sliced
- ½ teaspoon cinnamon

Instructions

1. Preheat oven to 225°F (110°C) and line a baking sheet with parchment paper.
2. Arrange apple slices in a single layer and sprinkle with cinnamon.

3. Bake for 2 hours, flipping halfway through, until crisp.
4. Let cool completely before serving.

Cooking Tips

- Store in an airtight container to keep them crisp.
- Use a mandoline slicer for even slices.

Health Benefits

- **Apples** provide fiber and help with digestion.
- **Cinnamon** supports blood sugar regulation and has anti-inflammatory properties.

---

15. Roasted Bell Peppers with Goat Cheese

A flavorful and nutritious snack with a creamy texture.

Servings: 2
Prep Time: 10 minutes
Cook Time: 15 minutes
Total Time: 25 minutes

Nutrition Per Serving

- **Calories:** 130
- **Protein:** 5g
- **Carbohydrates:** 10g
- **Fiber:** 3g
- **Fat:** 8g
- **Sodium:** 75mg

Ingredients

- 1 red bell pepper, sliced
- 2 tablespoons goat cheese
- 1 teaspoon olive oil
- ¼ teaspoon black pepper

Instructions

1. Preheat oven to 375°F (190°C).
2. Toss bell pepper slices with olive oil and black pepper.
3. Roast for 15 minutes until tender.
4. Top with crumbled goat cheese before serving.

Cooking Tips

Health Benefits

- **Bell peppers** are rich in vitamin C, which supports joint health.
- **Goat cheese** provides calcium for bone strength.

16. Warm Pear Compote with Walnuts (Limit walnuts)

A naturally sweet and cozy snack with heart-healthy fats.

Servings: 2
Prep Time: 5 minutes
Cook Time: 10 minutes
Total Time: 15 minutes

Nutrition Per Serving

- **Calories:** 150
- **Protein:** 2g
- **Carbohydrates:** 22g
- **Fiber:** 4g
- **Fat:** 6g
- **Sodium:** 5mg

Ingredients

- 1 ripe pear, diced
- 1 tablespoon chopped walnuts (limit portions)
- ½ teaspoon cinnamon
- 1 teaspoon honey

Instructions

1. In a small pan, cook diced pear over medium heat for 5 minutes.
2. Stir in cinnamon and honey, and cook for another 5 minutes until soft.
3. Remove from heat and sprinkle with walnuts before serving.

Cooking Tips

- Serve warm or chilled.
- Substitute walnuts with almonds for variation.

Health Benefits

- **Pears** aid digestion and provide hydration.
- **Walnuts (in moderation)** contain omega-3s that help reduce inflammation.

---

17. Butternut Squash and Almond Smoothie

A creamy, vitamin-rich smoothie perfect for a mid-day energy boost.

Servings: 1
Prep Time: 5 minutes
Total Time: 5 minutes

Nutrition Per Serving

- **Calories:** 180
- **Protein:** 4g

- **Carbohydrates:** 28g
- **Fiber:** 5g
- **Fat:** 6g
- **Sodium:** 20mg

Ingredients

- ½ cup cooked butternut squash
- ½ banana
- 1 tablespoon almond butter
- ½ teaspoon cinnamon
- ¾ cup unsweetened almond milk

Instructions

1. Blend all ingredients together until smooth.
2. Serve immediately.

Cooking Tips

- Add a few ice cubes for a chilled version.
- Substitute almond milk with oat milk for variety.

Health Benefits

- **Butternut squash** is rich in beta-carotene, which supports immune health.

18. Herb-Roasted Kale Chips

A crunchy, nutrient-packed snack with anti-inflammatory properties.

Servings: 2
Prep Time: 5 minutes
Cook Time: 15 minutes
Total Time: 20 minutes

Nutrition Per Serving

- **Calories:** 70
- **Protein:** 3g
- **Carbohydrates:** 10g
- **Fiber:** 2g
- **Fat:** 3g
- **Sodium:** 30mg

Ingredients

- 2 cups kale, washed and dried
- 1 teaspoon olive oil
- ½ teaspoon garlic powder
- ¼ teaspoon sea salt

Instructions

1. Preheat oven to 300°F (150°C).
2. Tear kale leaves into bite-sized pieces and toss with olive oil, garlic powder, and salt.

3. Spread in a single layer on a baking sheet.

4. Bake for 12–15 minutes until crispy.

Cooking Tips

- Watch closely to prevent burning.
- Sprinkle with nutritional yeast for a cheesy flavor.

Health Benefits

- **Kale** is packed with vitamins A, C, and K for joint health.
- **Garlic powder** has anti-inflammatory properties.

CHAPTER 8: 28-DAY MEAL PLAN FOR GOUT RELIEF

Day 1

- **Breakfast**: Quinoa Porridge with Blueberries and Almonds
- **Mid-Morning Snack**: Carrot and Hummus Sticks (Limit hummus portion)
- **Lunch**: Roasted Sweet Potatoes with Garlic & Steamed Green Beans
- **Afternoon Snack**: Baked Apple Chips with Cinnamon
- **Dinner**: Lemon Lentil Soup (Limit lentils to ½ cup per serving)

Day 2

- **Breakfast**: Avocado and Tomato on Whole-Grain Toast
- **Mid-Morning Snack**: Cucumber and Avocado Roll-Ups
- **Lunch**: Kale and Sweet Potato Stew
- **Afternoon Snack**: Frozen Banana and Almond Butter Bites
- **Dinner**: Butternut Squash and Apple Soup

Day 3

- **Breakfast**: Warm Oatmeal with Sliced Pears and Chia Seeds
- **Mid-Morning Snack**: Quinoa Crackers with Guacamole
- **Lunch**: Zucchini and Leek Soup with Whole-Grain Bread
- **Afternoon Snack**: Almond Butter and Apple Slices
- **Dinner**: Roasted Brussels Sprouts with Lemon & Tomato and Bell Pepper Salad

Day 4

- **Breakfast**: Pumpkin and Coconut Milk Smoothie
- **Mid-Morning Snack**: Herb-Roasted Kale Chips
- **Lunch**: Quinoa and Kale Salad with Citrus Dressing
- **Afternoon Snack**: Coconut Yogurt with Chia Seeds
- **Dinner**: Slow-Cooked Tomato and Quinoa Stew

Day 5

- **Breakfast**: Scrambled Eggs with Sautéed Spinach and Whole-Grain Toast
- **Mid-Morning Snack**: Zucchini Chips with Paprika
- **Lunch**: Warm Beet and Walnut Salad (Limit walnuts)
- **Afternoon Snack**: Baked Sweet Potato Fries
- **Dinner**: Mushroom-Free Vegetable Barley Soup

Day 6

- **Breakfast**: Butternut Squash and Almond Smoothie
- **Mid-Morning Snack**: Steamed Edamame with Sea Salt (Limit to ½ cup)
- **Lunch**: Cucumber and Avocado Salad with Lemon Dressing
- **Afternoon Snack**: Carrot and Ginger Energy Bites
- **Dinner**: Broccoli and Almond Soup

Day 7

- **Breakfast**: Whole-Grain Pancakes with Sliced Apples
- **Mid-Morning Snack**: Roasted Bell Peppers with Goat Cheese
- **Lunch**: Carrot and Apple Slaw with Quinoa Crackers
- **Afternoon Snack**: Warm Pear Compote with Walnuts (Limit walnuts)
- **Dinner**: Hearty Quinoa and Vegetable Stew

Day 8

- **Breakfast**: Overnight Oats with Pear and Almonds
- **Mid-Morning Snack**: Baked Apple Chips with Cinnamon
- **Lunch**: Roasted Sweet Potatoes with Garlic & Steamed Green Beans
- **Afternoon Snack**: Coconut Yogurt with Chia Seeds
- **Dinner**: Grilled Zucchini with Lemon Dressing & Quinoa

Day 9

- **Breakfast**: Zucchini and Goat Cheese Omelet
- **Mid-Morning Snack**: Quinoa Crackers with Guacamole
- **Lunch**: Carrot and Apple Slaw with Almond Dressing

- ✅ **Afternoon Snack**: Frozen Banana and Almond Butter Bites
- ✅ **Dinner**: Butternut Squash and Kale Risotto

Day 10

- ✅ **Breakfast**: Scrambled Egg Whites with Roasted Vegetables
- ✅ **Mid-Morning Snack**: Roasted Chickpeas with Turmeric (Limit to ½ cup)
- ✅ **Lunch**: Cabbage Slaw with Apple Cider Dressing & Quinoa
- ✅ **Afternoon Snack**: Almond Butter and Apple Slices
- ✅ **Dinner**: Zucchini and Sweet Potato Casserole

Day 11

- ✅ **Breakfast**: Pumpkin and Cinnamon Breakfast Muffins
- ✅ **Mid-Morning Snack**: Herb-Roasted Kale Chips
- ✅ **Lunch**: Steamed Carrot and Green Pea Salad
- ✅ **Afternoon Snack**: Steamed Edamame with Sea Salt (Limit to ½ cup)
- ✅ **Dinner**: Pan-Seared Tofu with Sesame Greens

Day 12

- ✅ **Breakfast**: Buckwheat Pancakes with Warm Berry Compote
- ✅ **Mid-Morning Snack**: Cucumber and Avocado Roll-Ups
- ✅ **Lunch**: Chickpea and Tomato Curry (Limit chickpeas) with Brown Rice
- ✅ **Afternoon Snack**: Carrot and Ginger Energy Bites
- ✅ **Dinner**: Herb-Roasted White Fish with Quinoa

Day 13

- ✅ **Breakfast**: Carrot and Apple Oatmeal Bowl
- ✅ **Mid-Morning Snack**: Roasted Bell Peppers with Goat Cheese
- ✅ **Lunch**: Warm Beet and Walnut Salad (Limit walnuts)
- ✅ **Afternoon Snack**: Coconut Yogurt with Chia Seeds
- ✅ **Dinner**: Tomato and Herb Stew with Quinoa

Day 14

☑ **Breakfast**: Warm Lemon and Ginger Detox Tea with Whole-Grain Toast

☑ **Mid-Morning Snack**: Zucchini Chips with Paprika

☑ **Lunch**: Roasted Pumpkin and Kale Salad

☑ **Afternoon Snack**: Baked Sweet Potato Fries

☑ **Dinner**: Slow-Cooked Tomato and Quinoa Soup

Day 15

☑ **Breakfast**: Turmeric-Spiced Golden Smoothie

☑ **Mid-Morning Snack**: Carrot and Hummus Sticks (Limit hummus portions)

☑ **Lunch**: Green Goddess Quinoa Bowl

☑ **Afternoon Snack**: Baked Apple Chips with Cinnamon

☑ **Dinner**: Zucchini and Spinach Whole-Grain Pasta (Spinach in moderation)

Day 16

☑ **Breakfast**: Almond Butter and Chia Toast on Whole-Grain Bread

☑ **Mid-Morning Snack**: Roasted Brussels Sprouts with Lemon (Limit to ½ cup)

☑ **Lunch**: Broccoli and Almond Stir-Fry

☑ **Afternoon Snack**: Pumpkin Seed Trail Mix (Limit portions)

☑ **Dinner**: Grilled Eggplant with Garlic Yogurt Sauce

Day 17

☑ **Breakfast**: Overnight Oats with Pear and Almonds

☑ **Mid-Morning Snack**: Cucumber and Avocado Roll-Ups

☑ **Lunch**: Tomato and Bell Pepper Salad with Olive Oil

☑ **Afternoon Snack**: Frozen Banana and Almond Butter Bites

☑ **Dinner**: Baked Lemon Chicken with Steamed Vegetables

Day 18

☑ **Breakfast**: Quinoa and Banana Breakfast Porridge

☑ **Mid-Morning Snack**: Quinoa Crackers with Guacamole

☑ **Lunch**: Zucchini Noodles with Basil Almond Pesto

☑ **Afternoon Snack**: Roasted Chickpeas

with Turmeric (Limit to ½ cup)

- [x] **Dinner**: Low-Purine Vegetable Stir-Fry with Brown Rice

Day 19

- [x] **Breakfast**: Coconut Yogurt with Chia and Flaxseeds
- [x] **Mid-Morning Snack**: Carrot and Ginger Energy Bites
- [x] **Lunch**: Steamed Cabbage with Olive Oil and Lemon Dressing
- [x] **Afternoon Snack**: Warm Pear Compote with Walnuts (Limit walnuts)
- [x] **Dinner**: Herb-Roasted White Fish with Quinoa

Day 20

- [x] **Breakfast**: Pumpkin and Cinnamon Breakfast Muffins
- [x] **Mid-Morning Snack**: Roasted Bell Peppers with Goat Cheese
- [x] **Lunch**: Zucchini and Sweet Potato Casserole
- [x] **Afternoon Snack**: Herb-Roasted Kale Chips
- [x] **Dinner**: Roasted Zucchini and Quinoa Pilaf

Day 21

- [x] **Breakfast**: Warm Cinnamon Quinoa with Berries
- [x] **Mid-Morning Snack**: Steamed Edamame with Sea Salt (Limit to ½ cup)
- [x] **Lunch**: Carrot and Parsnip Mash with Steamed Green Beans
- [x] **Afternoon Snack**: Homemade Quinoa Granola Bars
- [x] **Dinner**: Slow-Cooked Tomato and Quinoa Soup

Day 22

- [x] **Breakfast**: Flaxseed and Banana Energy Muffins
- [x] **Mid-Morning Snack**: Zucchini Chips with Paprika
- [x] **Lunch**: Cucumber and Cottage Cheese Stuffed Peppers
- [x] **Afternoon Snack**: Baked Sweet Potato Fries
- [x] **Dinner**: Baked Cod with Lemon and Herbs

Day 23

- **Breakfast**: Papaya and Coconut Breakfast Shake
- **Mid-Morning Snack**: Cucumber and Avocado Roll-Ups
- **Lunch**: Butternut Squash and Kale Side Dish with Quinoa
- **Afternoon Snack**: Almond Butter and Apple Slices
- **Dinner**: Chickpea and Tomato Curry (Chickpeas in moderation)

Day 24

- **Breakfast**: Scrambled Egg Whites with Roasted Vegetables
- **Mid-Morning Snack**: Steamed Green Beans with Almonds
- **Lunch**: Cabbage and White Bean Soup (Limit white beans to ½ cup)
- **Afternoon Snack**: Baked Apple Chips with Cinnamon
- **Dinner**: Grilled Zucchini with Lemon Dressing

Day 25

- **Breakfast**: Warm Lemon and Ginger Detox Tea with Whole-Grain Toast
- **Mid-Morning Snack**: Roasted Brussels Sprouts and Almond Salad (Limit to ½ cup per serving)
- **Lunch**: Tomato and Herb Stew with Quinoa
- **Afternoon Snack**: Carrot and Hummus Sticks (Limit hummus portions)
- **Dinner**: Roasted Sweet Potatoes with Garlic

Day 26

- **Breakfast**: Zucchini and Goat Cheese Omelet
- **Mid-Morning Snack**: Homemade Quinoa Granola Bars
- **Lunch**: Kale and Sweet Potato Stew
- **Afternoon Snack**: Herb-Roasted Kale Chips
- **Dinner**: Pan-Seared Tofu with Sesame Greens

Day 27

- **Breakfast**: Pumpkin and Cinnamon Breakfast Muffins
- **Mid-Morning Snack**: Cucumber and Avocado Salad with Lemon Dressing
- **Lunch**: Warm Beet and Goat Cheese

Salad

☑ **Afternoon Snack**: Frozen Banana and Almond Butter Bites

☑ **Dinner**: Sweet Potato and Carrot Mash with Grilled Vegetables

Day 28

☑ **Breakfast**: Spinach and Goat Cheese Scramble (Spinach in moderation)

☑ **Mid-Morning Snack**: Roasted Chickpeas with Turmeric (Limit to ½ cup)

☑ **Lunch**: Butternut Squash and Apple Soup

☑ **Afternoon Snack**: Carrot and Ginger Energy Bites

☑ **Dinner**: Slow-Cooked Tomato and Quinoa Soup

🛒 Week 1 Grocery Shopping List

Fruits & Vegetables

☑ Apples (3)

☑ Bananas (3)

☑ Avocado (2)

☑ Blueberries (1 cup)

☑ Carrots (6)

☑ Cucumbers (2)

☑ Zucchini (3)

☑ Kale (1 bunch)

☑ Spinach (1 small bag)

☑ Bell peppers (3, mixed colors)

☑ Brussels sprouts (1 cup)

☑ Tomatoes (3)

☑ Sweet potatoes (3)

☑ Pumpkin (1 small)

☑ Beets (2)

☑ Lemon (2)

☑ Garlic (3 cloves)

☑ Ginger (1 small piece)

Grains & Legumes

☑ Quinoa (2 cups)

☑ Brown rice (1 cup)

☑ Whole-grain bread (1 loaf)

☑ Oatmeal (1 cup)

☑ Chia seeds (½ cup)

☑ Almond flour (for muffins)

Proteins & Dairy

☑ White fish fillets (2)

☑ Chicken breast (1 large)

☑ Eggs (6)

☑ Goat cheese (½ cup)

☑ Greek yogurt (for sauce)

Nuts & Seeds

- [x] Almonds (½ cup)
- [x] Pumpkin seeds (¼ cup)
- [x] Walnuts (¼ cup, limited)

Pantry & Seasonings

- [x] Olive oil (1 bottle)
- [x] Cinnamon (1 small jar)
- [x] Turmeric (1 small jar)
- [x] Sea salt (as needed)

🛒 Week 2 Grocery Shopping List

Fruits & Vegetables

- [x] Apples (3)
- [x] Bananas (3)
- [x] Avocado (2)
- [x] Blueberries (1 cup)
- [x] Strawberries (1 cup)
- [x] Carrots (6)
- [x] Cucumbers (2)
- [x] Zucchini (3)
- [x] Kale (1 bunch)
- [x] Spinach (1 small bag)
- [x] Bell peppers (3, mixed colors)
- [x] Brussels sprouts (1 cup)
- [x] Tomatoes (3)
- [x] Sweet potatoes (3)
- [x] Butternut squash (1 small)
- [x] Beets (2)
- [x] Lemon (2)
- [x] Garlic (3 cloves)
- [x] Ginger (1 small piece)
- [x] Green beans (1 cup)

Grains & Legumes

- [x] Quinoa (2 cups)
- [x] Brown rice (1 cup)
- [x] Whole-grain pasta (1 cup)
- [x] Oatmeal (1 cup)
- [x] Chia seeds (½ cup)
- [x] Lentils (½ cup, limited)

Proteins & Dairy

- [x] White fish fillets (2)
- [x] Chicken breast (1 large)
- [x] Eggs (6)
- [x] Cottage cheese (½ cup)
- [x] Goat cheese (½ cup)
- [x] Greek yogurt (for sauce)

Nuts & Seeds

- [x] Almonds (½ cup)
- [x] Pumpkin seeds (¼ cup)
- [x] Walnuts (¼ cup, limited)

Pantry & Seasonings

- ☑ Olive oil (1 bottle)
- ☑ Cinnamon (1 small jar)
- ☑ Turmeric (1 small jar)
- ☑ Sea salt (as needed)
- ☑ Apple cider vinegar (for dressing)

🛒 **Week 3 Grocery Shopping List**

Fruits & Vegetables

- ☑ Apples (3)
- ☑ Pears (2)
- ☑ Bananas (3)
- ☑ Avocado (2)
- ☑ Blueberries (1 cup)
- ☑ Carrots (6)
- ☑ Cucumbers (2)
- ☑ Zucchini (3)
- ☑ Kale (1 bunch)
- ☑ Spinach (1 small bag)
- ☑ Bell peppers (3, mixed colors)
- ☑ Brussels sprouts (1 cup)
- ☑ Tomatoes (3)
- ☑ Sweet potatoes (3)
- ☑ Butternut squash (1 small)
- ☑ Beets (2)
- ☑ Lemon (2)
- ☑ Garlic (3 cloves)
- ☑ Ginger (1 small piece)
- ☑ Green beans (1 cup)

Grains & Legumes

- ☑ Quinoa (2 cups)
- ☑ Brown rice (1 cup)
- ☑ Whole-grain pasta (1 cup)
- ☑ Oatmeal (1 cup)
- ☑ Chia seeds (½ cup)
- ☑ Lentils (½ cup, limited)
- ☑ Chickpeas (½ cup, limited)

Proteins & Dairy

- ☑ White fish fillets (2)
- ☑ Chicken breast (1 large)
- ☑ Eggs (6)
- ☑ Cottage cheese (½ cup)
- ☑ Goat cheese (½ cup)
- ☑ Greek yogurt (for sauce)

Nuts & Seeds

- ☑ Almonds (½ cup)
- ☑ Pumpkin seeds (¼ cup)
- ☑ Walnuts (¼ cup, limited)

Pantry & Seasonings

- ☑ Olive oil (1 bottle)
- ☑ Cinnamon (1 small jar)

- ☑ Turmeric (1 small jar)
- ☑ Sea salt (as needed)
- ☑ Apple cider vinegar (for dressing)
- ☑ Tahini (for hummus)

🛒 Week 4 Grocery Shopping List

Fruits & Vegetables

- ☑ Apples (3)
- ☑ Pears (2)
- ☑ Bananas (3)
- ☑ Avocado (2)
- ☑ Blueberries (1 cup)
- ☑ Carrots (6)
- ☑ Cucumbers (2)
- ☑ Zucchini (3)
- ☑ Kale (1 bunch)
- ☑ Spinach (1 small bag)
- ☑ Bell peppers (3, mixed colors)
- ☑ Brussels sprouts (1 cup)
- ☑ Tomatoes (3)
- ☑ Sweet potatoes (3)
- ☑ Butternut squash (1 small)
- ☑ Beets (2)
- ☑ Lemon (2)
- ☑ Garlic (3 cloves)
- ☑ Ginger (1 small piece)
- ☑ Green beans (1 cup)

Grains & Legumes

- ☑ Quinoa (2 cups)
- ☑ Brown rice (1 cup)
- ☑ Whole-grain pasta (1 cup)
- ☑ Oatmeal (1 cup)
- ☑ Chia seeds (½ cup)
- ☑ Lentils (½ cup, limited)
- ☑ Chickpeas (½ cup, limited)

Proteins & Dairy

- ☑ White fish fillets (2)
- ☑ Chicken breast (1 large)
- ☑ Eggs (6)
- ☑ Cottage cheese (½ cup)
- ☑ Goat cheese (½ cup)
- ☑ Greek yogurt (for sauce)

Nuts & Seeds

- ☑ Almonds (½ cup)
- ☑ Pumpkin seeds (¼ cup)
- ☑ Walnuts (¼ cup, limited)

Pantry & Seasonings

- ☑ Olive oil (1 bottle)
- ☑ Cinnamon (1 small jar)
- ☑ Turmeric (1 small jar)

CONCLUSION

Managing gout isn't just about following a diet, it's about making consistent, mindful choices that support your body's health and well-being. The journey to a gout-free life requires patience, dedication, and an understanding of what works best for your body.

This cookbook has provided you with a wide variety of delicious, low-purine recipes designed to help reduce uric acid levels, prevent painful flare-ups, and improve your overall quality of life. By incorporating these meals into your daily routine, you can take control of your health while still enjoying flavorful and satisfying dishes.

The key to success is balance. While diet plays a crucial role, it is also important to embrace a holistic approach that includes hydration, exercise, and stress management. This combination will help you feel your best and maintain long-term gout relief.

Lifestyle Tips Beyond Diet: Exercise, Hydration, and Stress Management

While nutrition is the foundation of managing gout, there are additional lifestyle factors that significantly contribute to your overall well-being.

Here are some essential practices to support a gout-free life:

1. Stay Hydrated

💧 Water is essential for flushing excess uric acid from your body. Aim for at least **8–12 cups (2–3 liters) of water daily** to keep your kidneys functioning optimally. Herbal teas and infused water with lemon or cucumber can be great alternatives to plain water.

2. Maintain a Healthy Weight

⚖️ Excess weight can increase the risk of gout attacks. If needed, focus on gradual weight loss through balanced eating and regular physical activity. Avoid crash diets or extreme fasting, as these can actually trigger flare-ups.

3. Exercise Regularly

🏃 Engage in **low-impact exercises** such as walking, swimming, cycling, or yoga to improve circulation, strengthen joints, and maintain a healthy weight. High-impact activities may put stress on the joints, so listen to your body and choose movements that feel good.

4. Reduce Stress Levels

🧘 Stress can contribute to inflammation and worsen gout symptoms. Incorporate relaxation techniques such as meditation, deep breathing, journaling, or spending time in nature to lower stress and enhance overall well-being.

5. Get Enough Sleep

😴 Quality sleep is essential for reducing inflammation and supporting metabolic processes. Aim for **7–9 hours** of restful sleep each night. Establish a bedtime routine, limit screen time before bed, and create a relaxing environment to improve sleep quality.

6. Avoid Excess Alcohol and Sugary Drinks

🚫 Alcohol, especially beer and spirits, is high in purines and can significantly raise uric acid levels. Likewise, sugary drinks containing **high-fructose corn syrup** should be minimized. Stick to hydrating beverages like water, herbal teas, and homemade fruit-infused water.

How to Handle Occasional Flare-Ups

Despite your best efforts, occasional gout flare-ups may still occur. The key is to **act quickly** and implement relief strategies to reduce pain and inflammation.

1. Increase Water Intake

Drinking plenty of water helps flush out excess uric acid and can shorten the duration of a flare-up.

2. Rest and Elevate the Affected Joint

Avoid putting pressure on inflamed joints. Rest and keep the joint elevated to reduce swelling.

3. Apply Cold Therapy

Use an ice pack wrapped in a towel and apply it to the affected area for **15–20 minutes at a time** to help numb the pain and decrease inflammation.

4. Take Anti-Inflammatory Foods and Supplements

- **Cherries** (fresh or tart cherry juice)

- **Ginger tea** (anti-inflammatory properties)
- **Turmeric** (can be added to meals or taken as a supplement)

5. Avoid High-Purine and Trigger Foods

During a flare-up, avoid red meats, organ meats, seafood, alcohol, and processed foods to prevent worsening symptoms. Stick to a clean, whole-foods diet.

6. Speak with Your Doctor If Needed

If flare-ups become frequent or severe, consult a healthcare professional. Medications may be needed to manage uric acid levels effectively.

Healing and managing gout is a lifelong journey, but you have the power to take control of your health. By following the **low-purine recipes** in this cookbook, staying hydrated, exercising regularly, and managing stress, you are setting yourself up for long-term success.

Remember: **progress, not perfection.** You don't have to be perfect every day just make small, mindful choices that support your well-being.

Celebrate your victories, no matter how small. Every meal you choose wisely, every glass of water you drink, and every step you take towards a healthier lifestyle brings you closer to **pain-free living**.

You are not alone in this journey. Thousands of people have successfully managed their gout through diet and lifestyle changes, and so can you!

Stay committed, stay inspired, and enjoy the process of nourishing your body with delicious, healing foods. Wishing you health, happiness, and a **gout-free life!**

Share Your Thoughts

Thank you for taking the time to explore *The Ultimate Gout Diet Cookbook for Seniors*.

I sincerely hope this book has provided you with valuable knowledge, delicious recipes, and practical strategies to help you manage gout and enjoy a healthier, pain-free life.

If you found this cookbook helpful, I would truly appreciate it if you could take a moment to leave honest feedback on Amazon. Your feedback not only helps others who are looking for reliable gout-friendly meal solutions, but it also allows me to continue creating high-quality resources that make a difference in people's lives.

Your thoughts and experiences matter! A quick review can help others on their journey toward better health.

I'd love to hear from you! If you have any questions, success stories, or recipe suggestions, feel free to reach out. Your feedback and engagement inspire me to keep writing and sharing valuable content.

Thank you for being part of this journey. Wishing you health, happiness, and many delicious, gout-friendly meals ahead!

With gratitude,

Amelia Sharon

Printed in Great Britain
by Amazon